Volume 2

CONFLICTS IN THE NATIONAL HEALTH SERVICE

CONFLICTS IN THE NATIONAL HEALTH SERVICE

Edited by
KEITH BARNARD
and
KENNETH LEE

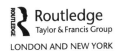

Routledge
Taylor & Francis Group

LONDON AND NEW YORK

First published in 1977 by Croom Helm Ltd.

This edition first published in 2022
by Routledge
4 Park Square, Milton Park, Abingdon, Oxon OX14 4RN

and by Routledge
605 Third Avenue, New York, NY 10158

Routledge is an imprint of the Taylor & Francis Group, an informa business

British Library Cataloguing in Publication Data
A catalogue record for this book is available from the British Library

ISBN: 978-0-367-52469-2 (Set)
ISBN: 978-1-032-25229-2 (Volume 2) (hbk)
ISBN: 978-1-032-25237-7 (Volume 2) (pbk)
ISBN: 978-1-003-28222-8 (Volume 2) (ebk)

DOI: 10.4324/9781003282228

Publisher's Note
The publisher has gone to great lengths to ensure the quality of this reprint but points out that some imperfections in the original copies may be apparent.

Disclaimer
The publisher has made every effort to trace copyright holders and would welcome correspondence from those they have been unable to trace.

Conflicts in the National Health Service

Edited by
KEITH BARNARD and KENNETH LEE

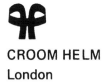

CROOM HELM
London

PRODIST
New York

© 1977 Keith Barnard and Kenneth Lee
Croom Helm Ltd, 2-10 St John's Road, London SW11

ISBN 0-85664-420-X

First published in the United States by
PRODIST
a division of
Neale Watson Academic Publications, Inc.
156 Fifth Avenue, New York 10010

Library of Congress Cataloging in Publication Data

Main entry under title:

Conflicts in the national health service.

    1. Great Britain – National Health Service. 2. Health
services administration – Great Britain. I. Barnard,
Keith. II. Lee, M. A.
RA412.5.G7C87 1977   362.1'0941   76-57740
ISBN 0-88202-114-1

Printed in Great Britain
by Redwood Burn Ltd, Trowbridge and Esher

CONTENTS

TABLES AND FIGURES

CONTRIBUTORS

Keith A. Barnard Deputy Director and Lecturer in Health Planning, Nuffield Centre for Health Services Studies, The University of Leeds

Stuart J. Dimmock Lecturer in Industrial Relations, Nuffield Centre for Health Services Studies, The University of Leeds

Mary Ann Elston Research Fellow, Nuffield Centre for Health Services Studies, The University of Leeds

Arthur Gunawardena Part-time Lecturer in Health Economics, Nuffield Centre for Health Services Studies, The University of Leeds

Chris J. Ham Research Assistant, Nuffield Centre for Health Services Studies, The University of Leeds

Malcolm L. Johnson Lecturer in Sociology, Nuffield Centre for Health Services Studies, The University of Leeds

Kenneth Lee Lecturer in Health Economics, Nuffield Centre for Health Services Studies, The University of Leeds

Andrew F. Long Lecturer in Quantitative Aspects of Management, Nuffield Centre for Health Services Studies, The University of Leeds

J. Crossley Sunderland Visiting Lecturer in Health Service Management, Nuffield Centre for Health Services Studies, The University of Leeds

David Towell Lecturer in Organisation Theory, Nuffield Centre for Health Services Studies, The University of Leeds

TO DONALD MACMILLAN

PREFACE

By the end of 1975, nearly two years after the official introduction of the reorganised National Health Service, it was apparent that the Service was beset by conflicts and tensions. Whatever the possible causes of this unrest the government of the day was moved to announce its decision to set up a Royal Commission—'To consider in the interests both of the patients and of those who work in the National Health Service the best use and management of the financial and manpower resources of the National Health Service.'

About that time, with the government's decision announced, the editors invited their colleagues as informed observers of the NHS to prepare a set of papers which would explore some of the most pressing problems besetting the Service. From their perspectives, largely as social scientists involved in the study of health services, they were invited to choose and develop their own themes. They were, however, encouraged to consult with one another in order to identify and develop the links between the themes and issues they selected. This collection of essays is the result of their individual and collective endeavours.

Inevitably the range of issues raised and perspectives offered are less than total; the general theme of this book necessarily reflects only those issues the writers find relevant to their consideration of the NHS. Readers will readily identify gaps in this catalogue of items on the NHS agenda. In deliberately settling for breadth of scope, it would still be foolish to make a pretence at either comprehensiveness or finality.

None the less, there is something to be said for reading the essays as a book. For the writers have addressed themselves to the prior task of identifying and clarifying some of the key conflicts and tensions in and facing the NHS; and with which the public, politicians and professionals will need to come to terms. In such a way it is hoped that the book will be of special interest not only to those working in the NHS but to all those who would modestly claim to be, or wish to be, students of the NHS and its practices.

In making our acknowledgements we must start by recording that each contributor to this collection wishes to own a debt to fellow contributors. While no corporate effort has been made to prepare a collective judgement and each author speaks for herself or himself, all have benefited from the mutual exchange of ideas and advice. They all wish to record the invaluable assistance of their secretaries in bringing typed order out of scarcely decipherable drafts. The editors wish particularly to acknowledge their own secretaries Mrs P. Hollick and Mrs S. Nutter, who have shouldered cheerfully a particularly heavy burden in preparing the complete text for publication. Our thanks are also prompted to our wives for their display of domestic patience as deadlines approached. Finally, the thanks of all contributors go out to other colleagues and to a countless number of individuals in and associated with the health field whose own ideas and experiences, revealed in our close contacts and co-operation with them, have contributed materially to our understanding of this field. In each case, however, the final form and ideas expressed in the papers must be, and are, the responsibility of the individual authors, and theirs alone.

Keith Barnard
October, 1976   Kenneth Lee

1 PROMISES, PATIENTS AND POLITICS: THE CONFLICTS OF THE NHS

Keith A. Barnard

I

This book is about problems. It is about problems which have surfaced, are surfacing, or are expected to surface. These problems have many causes, and indeed allow of several alternative explanations. But it is not unreasonable to see the roots of these problems in promises, patients and politics. Back in 1948, the public was led to believe that through the inauguration of a national health service, we could conquer at least one of Beveridge's Five Giants—that of Disease. That promise remains a mirage, yet expectations rise with every promise of a new breakthrough in medical science to relieve distress and defer death. And then again in 1974, the Service was subjected to a massive organisational upheaval and its whole administration put into the melting pot with the promise that while reorganisation was not about patient care, it would indirectly ensure better quality care. Time has passed and the promise is perceived as unfulfilled—certainly by staff and indeed by the public, at least through their proxies, the Community Health Councils. Thus, the problems of the Service can be seen to be, in an important measure, the problems of unfulfilled promises.

To the staff, the problems are not just promises, or receding promises, of adequate resources to do a good job for the public they serve. Patients too are a cause of anxiety, concern or even anger. The world of grateful patients, angelic nurses and learned doctors has long been confined between the covers of romantic fiction. Indeed the no-longer grateful patients are often likely to want to be equal partners in the determination of services. In contrast, other patients may now expect general practitioners to make decisions and take responsibility where an earlier generation would have used common sense, self-help, and had an intelligently circumscribed idea of what the doctor could be asked to do. Families may now even expect hospitals to relieve them of their responsibilities for their dependent members, the old and the mentally disordered. To add to these pressures from some sections of the public, patients are increasingly acting collectively to bring further influence to bear through pressure groups at both national and local level—a pressure, moreover, which can no longer be discounted.

To the observer the problems of the NHS are often seen as the problems of politics. In the cosy world of a decade or more ago, it was possible to sound plausible in pleading to keep politics out of health or health out of politics. But politics have rudely broken in. As in other sectors of public life, improvement in everything cannot be achieved by tomorrow. With the possible and the desirable always running ahead of both the resources available and the intellectual and emotional time and energy needed to harness those resources to provide a service, so enter problems of choice, of objectives and priorities, and of strategies to attain the desired ends. In short, so enters politics. These are matters for society acting through government and other political institutions, not least the health authorities. But government is dependent on those who provide the services even though the constitutional formal responsibility is government's.

So, equally, the politics of the organisation are as vital to those within the Service: how are they to order priorities within the organisation; how do they interpret government policies and exhortations; how do they respond to the pressures from the local community; how do they start to collaborate with other agencies providing caring services; and how do they respond to the ambitions and aspirations of their colleagues in seeking increased status and recognition as much as higher incomes? In summary: how are conflicts of interest and values acknowledged and handled on the local stage? Certainly, these political problems are emerging with greater intensity and the time seems past when these problems of the NHS could be claimed as soluble by the techniques of medical or economic or management science. Expert solutions always evade or conceal the underlying problem of politics— in a situation of choice, whose will prevails?

II

But before exploring these kinds of issues in the remainder of the book, and because so much is expected of and claimed for the NHS by both protagonists and antagonists alike, it might be worthwhile to look at the NHS *in the simplest terms:* how it is structured; what has influenced its development, and, to some extent, how it relates to the rest of society. More detailed discussion on particular matters will follow from later contributors.

In the first place, the NHS is essentially a system of medical care, with access to the system almost invariably initiated by self-referral to a general medical practitioner. Ideally, there is a continuing relationship between the individual and the general practitioner who thereby acquires a comprehensive understanding of the individual, his health status and needs. The practitioner is the decision-maker as to what further resources available under the NHS should be made available to the individual, e.g. by prescribing drugs or by referring him to hospital for a specialist consultation. In this latter case, the hospital consultant acquires responsibility for the individual's medical care, but surrenders this back to the GP at the end of the particular episode of care and treatment.

This system of care functions in the context of an organisational structure. The structure of the NHS when it was set up in 1948 was essentially the culmination of an historical evolution of hospital provision, medical professional practice, and public administration, together with a number of compromises necessary to acquire the maximum political consensus that would enable the Service to be launched. The effect of the decisions made on structure was to create three administrative sectors providing, respectively, general practitioner services, hospital and specialist services, and, thirdly, a range of community and personal support services as diverse as home nursing and ambulances.

This tripartite structure was soon seen to have problems. Although the service was financed by public expenditure, mainly from general taxation, the administrative fragmentation made co-ordination of services and 'rational' planning very difficult. Pressure grew by the 1960s for some form of administrative unification to facilitate co-ordination and comprehensive planning better in order to ensure better quality patient care. Various proposals were subjected to public debate and eventually in 1973 Parliament passed the legislation authorising the re-organisation of the NHS.

As under the original NHS Act, 1946, the Secretary of State for Social Services was ultimately responsible for the NHS; through the Department of Health and Social Security (DHSS) he would issue policy guidelines to the Service and would make financial allocations to the 14 Regional Health Authorities (RHAs) who, in turn, would act similarly towards the 90 Area Health Authorities (AHAs), within their territory. For management purposes large Areas were divided into comprehensive Health Districts, resulting in the creation of about 200 such Districts in England and Wales. The boundaries of the Area Health Authorities were fixed to be coterminous with the new local authorities — principally the county councils (in the conurbations, with the metropolitan district councils and, in London, with groupings of boroughs). Although the AHAs were constitutionally quite separate from local government, they had an obligation to collaborate with their matching councils over matters of joint concern and, in particular, were expected to plan together those services, such as the care of the elderly, where their contributions were complementary. Two other features of the new structure were the provision of professional advisory committees at Regional and Area levels to enable the views of the medical and other health professions to be made known to the Authority before decisions were made, and at District level, a District Medical Committee, representing all medical practitioners, would be an important influence on the District management team.

At the same time, it was recognised that the consumer voice was also needed as an influence on the Area Authority and on District management. A Community Health Council was established in each District to act as a public watchdog, patients' friend, and constructively critical commentator on the Service's plans and performance. For the first time there was an attempt to create a consumer voice identifiably separate from management to match the voice of the professional providers of services which had always been heard.

The momentum for reorganisation of the NHS which built up from the mid-1960s coincided with certain trends that were to become influential in the NHS. First, there was a world-wide growth of interest in health planning and organisation reflected in the professional literature on medical care and in the expert publications of the World Health Organisation. In essence, the planning argument was that socio-economic development could not be left to chance and that the health sector was an important element which needed to be integrated into overall social planning. A number of particular factors were identified, including the pressure on human and financial resources, the growing technological possibilities thrown up by medical science and by engineering, increased consumer expectations, and the general political pressure to provide health services that accorded with the perceived needs of the population. Against that background, a participative form of planning involving all the interested parties—consumers, professional providers, administrators and politicians—was seen as a way of generating realistic proposals for the future commanding widespread commitment to their successful implementation. In this sense, planning was seen as much as a broad-based political and social process as a set of technical and administrative procedures that could be remitted to a designated set of professional experts.

A second trend was the growing commitment of large organisations (initially in the private sector and later spreading to the public sector) to some form of corporate strategy and management. Studies have shown that many large organisations were influenced by a recurring set of factors: the complexity of the organisation in both its internal and external relationships; the very size of the enterprise; the sensitivity of the organisation and its business to technological change; and the importance of capital developments to the enterprise. By any of the conventional criteria, e.g. the size of its operating budget, its number of employees, its number of operational locations, or its number of agents, the NHS is a very large organisation and demonstrates in some significant measure the same kinds of influences that have led other large enterprises to adopt the corporate approach.

With all modern technologically-based organisations too much is at stake to be left to chance. There must be some attempt to minimise uncertainty, 'to control the future'. The size factor makes it increasingly difficult to control the enterprise from the centre, from head office. A way must be found of identifying the key decisions whereby the centre can control the general direction and development of the whole organisation while delegating as much operational decision-making as possible to the subsidiary units who can act both in the light of centrally-determined general policy and in their awareness of local conditions and circumstances. A formal corporate planning and management system is seen as an effective means of achieving this. Each subsidiary agrees plans with headquarters, who then authorise the subsidiary's expenditure and monitor the performance and issue the instructions for corrective action should this become necessary. Thus, broad policy and financial control remains with the centre who are also relieved of a good deal of detailed decision-making that for various reasons they are not fitted to discharge.

Given the apparent appropriateness of this model for the NHS, it is not surprising that once the structure of statutory authorities for the reorganised NHS was fixed, and the objective of integrating the services to provide better patient care was reaffirmed, attention was directed towards evolving a corporate planning system; designed to achieve that objective, and to enable the operational relationships between the various tiers in the structure (government, region, area, district) to be developed as free of friction as possible.

There are, however, a number of problems in applying the model to the NHS which need to be identified and which will no doubt influence the way the corporate approach in the NHS finally evolves. There is no simple product, or indeed range of products, the manufacture of which could be rationalised in the interests of efficiency. Nor do consumers of health services appear to behave with the same kind of rationality that they are assumed to display when making decisions about, say, household durables. Thirdly, the machinery for consultation and collaboration at the Area level with the consumers, the professional providers and the local authority may generate pressures on the AHA and their officers contrary to the guidance and, possibly, directives reaching the Area from government and the regional authority. Lastly, in emphasising planning, there is an assumption that one's present decision-making is decisively influenced by a wish to see a desirable state of affairs being reached at a point in the future: the culture of the Health Service and the medical profession emphasises relieving *present* problems of pain and distress rather than working towards some future benefit: moreover, the motivation of the politicians who temporarily occupy the highest posts as Ministers heading up the government department (DHSS) responsible for the Service, lies in the need to demonstrate their impact quickly if they are to further their political careers. In fact, there is a direct conflict between long-term planning and the pressures of the political arena. These are potentially powerful factors militating against the sustained application of the corporate planning approach as outlined here to the development of the NHS.

However, a system has now been introduced (from April 1976) and is being applied throughout the Service. The particular mechanisms used to achieve the balance between essential central control and delegated decision-making are complicated and need not be spelt out here for the essential principle is a simple one. The Secretary of State, through his Department, DHSS, issues policy guidelines and makes financial allocations. These are filtered through regional and area authorities to the managers and the staff providing the services. In return, the providers make proposals for developing and (particularly important in times of financial restraint) rationalising the services in the light of guidelines and the funds made available to them, and in the light of their awareness of the local situation, and their consultations with all local interests. In short, the system is an attempt to reconcile conflicting pressures which are indeed common to all public sector organisations—the need to introduce efficient management to husband limited resources; and at the same time to recognise that the organisation is operating in a political context and that means must be found to give open expression to conflicts of interests and values in order that they can be reconciled or accommodated in policy and decision-making.

For a long time the medical care field has been spared these pressures. Medical activity with its connotation of life-saving interventions was universally held to be self-evidently desirable and deserving of increasing resources. As its technological possibilities expanded, so did

public expectations and also the size of its financial and human resource budget. But gradually this view has come under pressure. A
number of informed commentators have questioned the efficacy of
medical interventions and have established that the dramatic improvements in health as measured by life expectancy and infant mortality
(the classic indicators) occurred before the explosion in high-cost,
high-technology, hospital-based medicine and that the dramatic growth
of the medical care budget (measured in constant prices to take account
of inflation) over the past twenty years has coincided with minimum
improvements in life expectancy. Thus, there are growing doubts being
expressed about the net benefit accruing from further investment in
high-technology medicine; and growing advocacy that future investment
should be directed to non-medical activities such as better housing,
better social support and income maintenance for the socially dis-
advantaged, and generally improving public amenities and the physical
environment. Parallel with this admittedly still fledgling assault on the
medical establishment is another attack on the way the NHS has evolved:
not only has high-technology medicine been favoured with resources at
the expense of the 'caring' specialties of geriatrics and psychiatry, but
gross geographical inequalities (measured on a population basis) have
been perpetuated and any mitigating efforts so far have proved ineffective. Thus, the corporate planners and managers have to effect a
reorientation both in geography and in the emphasis on service development. This exercise will be conducted in a climate of winners and losers
where the losers can be expected to be very vociferous and not without
political resources harnessed in an effort to minimise the impact of the
planned changes.

So far the picture has been painted of the NHS emerging as another
form of large-scale organisation or public corporation with its pressures
and contradictions, its search for efficiency and its attempts to accommodate its internal and external political environment. Above all,
conflicts and tensions will have emerged as increasing possibilities and
expectations compete with limited financial and human resources; and
as decisions to cut back on the increasing emphasis on high technology
in order to favour the caring services are perceived as attacks on all hospital services, even those whose efficacy has been conclusively
demonstrated.

III

Against that background sketch the course to be charted through the
rest of the book can now be plotted. Because the NHS is a system of

medical care, attention is first directed towards the medical profession, who have necessarily dominated the Service as their skills are crucial to its purpose. But the dominance of the medical profession and their high status in society at large may now be ebbing. For various reasons, their authority is being questioned and their own ranks, always in some senses divided, are now showing conflicts in a way that had not been expected until recently.

A consideration of the problems of the profession leads into the one essay which looks at a service provided to patients where the problems arise of what is rational and efficient, of how to reconcile apparently conflicting objectives, of what behaviour professionals have a right to expect of patients; and of what the implications are of taking patients' wishes and behaviour into account. The service examined is the Accident and Emergency Department, but the problems of patient access and efficient service reflect the problems facing much of the NHS generally.

Taking account of patient behaviour in their utilisation of A and E Departments in turn calls for a broadly based review of the patient—practitioner relationship. In view of the growing movement of consumerism in all sections of society and trading, it is not surprising that eventually this has made some impact on medical care. But through using the growing body of research findings from medical sociology, there are grounds for perceiving some fundamental changes taking place in the patient—doctor relationship. If these trends continue, the relationship will emerge more as one of partnership and will call for a significant reappraisal on the part of practitioners as to what they can expect from patients and how they should behave towards them. Clearly this is a radical position which is in some measure challenged by the next paper which looks at patients and their representatives as one of the power-holding parties in our pluralistic democracy. It looks at the ability of the Community Health Councils to exercise influence locally and national patient pressure groups' ability to influence government. The paper is not sanguine in its conclusions about collective patient power. The reader is left to weigh up the lessons of the analysis offered by both these papers.

If patients are seen as in a weak bargaining position, either in the consulting room or at the committee table, then traditionally so have hospital staff been seen. In particular, the supporting ancillary staff providing the so-called hotel services in hospitals were seemingly deferential and quite unaffected by the attempts of trade unions to organise them. The seventies have seen a radical change: ancillary workers are better organised; their leaders take overtly political stances on issues that bring them into conflict with both government and the erstwhile dominant medical profession; and, at a local level, they increasingly take industrial action. The evidence available suggests that the Department and Health Service managers have yet to come to terms with this significant change in the power structure.

This leads on to a view of the problems as seen by the administrator. The administrator may feel particularly threatened: the 'bureaucrat' is fair game to any critic firing from the left or the right. He is seen as having profited from reorganisation, both by an 'unwarranted' lift in his salary and by an enhancing of his power. Such a caricature misses the point: the administrator may be as opposed to, or, at the very least, as concerned about the new order as any other health worker. Reorganisation has made management more difficult especially where it matters, in the institutions providing services to patients. It could be argued that the elaborate machinery of team management has reduced his influence, not enhanced it, and without any compensating benefit in improved efficiency of service. He resents not only being identified with the system but also the readiness of other groups to take industrial action to enhance their power and incomes. When they take industrial action, he moves to ensure that the results of that action are inconvenience to management, not danger to patients. What would be the consequences if administrators finally exhausted their tolerance and patience with the aspirations of other groups, and took industrial action of their own? Who then would hold the organisation together, and for how long? To raise these questions is to suggest that the administrators' problems may have been seriously underestimated.

But the lay administrator is not the only manager with problems. On one reading of the reorganisation strategy, *the* key innovation was the emergence of community medicine as a crucial influence on the development of health services. The role of the District Community Physician was to be the means whereby an informed professional appraisal could be made of the *health problems* of the population and success of the *health services* in alleviating these problems. If better-quality integrated care meant anything, it meant this. How well has the DCP been able to respond to his challenge; how has he been able to cope with his legacy of not being a clinician; has he been able to act as the intermediary between the services and the community? Has he been able to exert any influence on realigning the development of the Service? These questions are, of course, partly rhetorical, and their implications are that more efforts are needed from many quarters to support community medicine as it grows into an effective role; and the lesson for the Community Physicians is that they must not lose sight of the purpose for which their posts were created.

But if the DCP is charged with introducing a scientific element into service planning and development, what are the realities behind the concept of rational decision-making? Taking as its case material population forecasts and projections—essential raw material in the DCP's 'new epidemiology' and population medicine—the penultimate paper looks at the limitations of forecasting, the conceptual problems and the practical difficulties and concludes that ultimately, decision-making rests on judgement—judgement as to the inherent plausibility of the assumptions behind the scientific calculations, and the intuition of the decision-maker as to the consequences of his decision. The positive lesson emerges that for informed debate between interested parties, it is essential that the assumptions are always made explicit.

By way of conclusion, the final paper returns to the inevitability of rationing, choice and political judgement. Given the euphoric sentiments expressed and believed at the time the NHS was launched, the reality is now to be seen in somewhat different terms. In the first place, calls on public expenditure have not declined as the founding fathers clearly expected; the prevalence of sickness and the evidence of waiting lists are as visible today as they were in Aneurin Bevan's time. The art of political judgement in deciding how much money should be devoted to the NHS—and in what directions—is a topic currently generating a good deal of copy for both journals and conference platforms. The crucial question at the heart of the politics of the NHS is, then, who should be making these judgements? Of one thing we can be certain; no politician will be eager to sacrifice an opportunity to make his impact upon this debate for the sake of local democracy. Hence, the ideal of devolved responsibility in the NHS will repeatedly come up against the reality of centralisation at least for as long as the NHS remains in its present form; or indeed even if it were to become, in time, another function of local government.

IV

That then is the scope of this book. What thoughts and speculations might it prompt in the mind of the reader as the debate on our medical care gathers momentum? The initial reaction might well be that providers of medical care will be reluctant to accept that further expenditure in their sector of the service is not unquestionably justified. Members of the public, though they have not so far displayed much interest in the working of the NHS, may some day soon experience great anxiety if they are told that the services they 'need' are either not available or will only be available after inordinate, possibly fatal delay. How can the policy-makers, the planners and administrators respond to this situation?

One school of thought will look for a lowering of expectations on both sides. Intensive efforts could be made to establish and select those medical interventions which are proved to be effective and then take action to see that resources are equitably distributed to provide *effective* medical care. Both providers and consumers would then have to come to terms with the limits to medicine, though this change of expectations could only come about after an intensive education campaign of the profession and the public as to what constitutes rational behaviour in providing and seeking medical care. All this has the look of a counsel of perfection, providing little immediate guidance for those charged with preparing planning proposals for their areas and districts. It also raises further questions as to who shall judge what constitutes 'rational' and by what criteria?

Yet, what is the alternative? Is it the art of muddling on: continuing the time-honoured practices of marginal adjustments, making concessions, judging issues piecemeal, maintaining some semblance of stability and continuity? But while this is a probable scenario, it may be storing up trouble leading to an eventual breakdown of the Service. So, it could be argued, attention should focus on gradually improving the rationale of the Service, so that there is a framework for identifying objectives and strategies, and for developing criteria by which options or possible courses of action could be considered and adopted or rejected.

What form might this take? First, it could be argued that any change in the pattern of provision of services would only be considered if the prime purpose of the new activity relieved pain or distress and could be shown to be capable of doing that without making undue claims on resources. No priority would then be given to proposals directed at producing an alleged cure, particularly if it were for a numerically small group of the population. Likewise, all expensive procedures would be phased out as quickly as practicable enabling resources to be reallocated to relieve pain and distress. Now this rationale has a humanitarian ring, and tries to offer something to the whole population, but, it may be thought, pays insufficient attention to the contribution that the health sector should be making to the development of society as a whole.

This line of reasoning suggests a second approach: the medical care system could be directed to the economically productive elements of the population. In future, health services would be reconstructed to concentrate on such groups as the young and those of working age to ensure that they are brought to a peak of mental and physical fitness, on the basis that the future of the economy and indeed of the society rested with them. Of course, it might be felt that the argument sits too closely and comfortably with concepts of social Darwinism for it to be accepted by present-day society; especially as it appears to deny those humanitarian values that have traditionally underpinned our principles (though not always our practices) of caring for the feeble in mind and body.

This then brings us back to the start of the argument—to limit the provision of services to those of proven efficiency and, further, to submit any proposals for innovations in services to the most critical scrutiny. Only by following this rationale could value for money be guaranteed without having to make any invidious choice between groups in the population, because decisions would then be made on technical, not human, grounds.

If, however, it be thought that all these ways are too rigorous, too unbending, too inflexible to be turned into a set of genuine operating rules, might it then be just possible to attempt a consensual politics approach and, by extended consultation and discussion, agree that certain services were essential (e.g. environmental health, child health, maternity, accident and emergency) and that others, though desirable (e.g. transplant surgery, plastic surgery) would only be provided once the essential services were operating at an agreed acceptable level?

But is that too innocent a view? Certainly it is not too distantly removed from the approach currently being adopted. There is now an emphasis on published national priorities susceptible to change through feedback from the NHS through the planning system. There is a parallel, if so far muted, effort to interest the general public in prevention and positive health promotion. There is also evidence that health issues are being seen as involving more than the medically oriented health service, and that an interdepartmental and inter-agency collaborative approach is required. Yet intuitively one remains sceptical about the efficacy of present initiatives and intentions. It is to be hoped that evidence emerges to contradict that scepticism. In the meantime, one feels that there must first be a massive upsurge in enlightenment (and a matching denial of self-interest) among politicians, providers and patients, if the politics of goodwill and consensus are to pervade our medical care system. We can, of course, have the politics of negotiation—

in contradistinction to consensus—and perhaps we might start there. We should admit to paying more attention to the concepts of the incrementalists, of bargaining and mutual adjustment, to accommodate conflict.

This is a deliberately cautious reaction, offered as a starting point. The absence of obvious easy solutions must be the stimulus in the search for real understanding of the problems of providing medical care and promoting health in the population. The conventional wisdom, emphasising the rational approach and leading in the directions captured in the preceding paragraphs, is unlikely to be enough. We are not dealing with entirely rational phenomena, and there is nothing in our cultural, social and political history to suggest that the NHS and its objectives could ever be dealt with as a technical exercise. To go beyond received thinking is the task of the Royal Commission. Their report and the general reaction it generates must, when the time comes, be judged in this light.

2 MEDICAL AUTONOMY: CHALLENGE AND RESPONSE

Mary Ann Elston

Introduction

Since the mid-nineteenth century the British medical profession has established a position of great influence over all aspects of health care and in society as a whole.[1] This 'medical dominance' is being increasingly questioned from several directions and many doctors are expressing concern about where they may, or should, be going both as individual doctors and as an occupation. This paper will explore some of these challenges and their consequences for the medical profession.[2] The challenges discussed are primarily those from within the existing Health Service structures but the explanation of their origin must often be sought in the wider social context in which the National Health Service exists.

The significance of these challenges to 'medical dominance' arises from the prevailing medical view that freedom to control their own work and the work of others involved in the provision of health services is a 'necessary condition for the proper performance of work'.[3] Any challenges to the medical profession's established position are responded to in terms of the threat to professional or clinical freedom. In 1946 the British Medical Association's opposition to the establishment of the NHS was couched in these terms and, as many commentators have pointed out, the NHS has increased rather than threatened the independence of the medical profession.[4] At the time of writing (September 1976) there is concern over 'the greatest threat to the independence of the medical profession since the controversy associated with the NHS thirty years ago': the Labour government's Bill to phase out private medicine facilities from the NHS.[5]

Discontent amongst doctors is not a new phenomenon nor confined to the era of the NHS,[6] but the present situation is one in which doctors, like all members of society, have seen their standards of living affected by inflation and consequent pressure for change both from within their own ranks and from outside. The 'paybeds' issue is just one manifestation of a complex of underlying conflicts between sectors of the profession; between doctors and other health workers; and between the profession and the state. The central concern of this paper is not with value judgements about the challenges, but with the fact that they have been made at all. For this in itself indicates a shift in the balance of power away from the medical profession, even if to date for the most part, the attacks have been resisted.

The first challenge considered comes from within medicine itself and from changes in the population and the morbidity patterns doctors are called upon to treat. These are such that the effectiveness and the efficiency of much of modern medicine is being questioned. This, in turn, has consequences for the established structure of the profession and the allocation of resources to different sectors of the health services. Secondly, and following from both this first change and changes outside medicine, the doctor's right to control the work of other groups, and, on occasion, his own work, is being questioned by other Health Service workers and by patients.[7] The third area of change considered is within the profession itself. Here the challenge is not so much to the autonomy of the profession as a whole but to the established leadership's ability to represent the real interests of its members. All these challenges have repercussions on the relationship between the profession and the state.[8]

The relationship between the profession and the state is of central importance in the analysis of professional autonomy and dominance.[9] Freidson, a leading American medical sociologist, has summarised the relationship in this way:

> The foundation of medicine's control over its work is. . . clearly *political* in character, involving the aid of the state in establishing and maintaining the profession's pre-eminence. . . it is by the interaction between formal agents or agencies of the occupation and officials of the state that the occupation's control over its work is established and shaped.[10] (emphasis added)

It is evident that the explanation for the dominant position of the medical profession must be sought in an analysis of the organisation and power in society and in the relationship with the state of this occupational group rather than solely in the inherent nature of the work.[11] Thus, 'professionalisation' is a *process* by which some occupations have achieved autonomy through state recognition of monopoly of the provision of a particular service. The point is well illustrated by the successful campaign for registration leading to the 1858 Medical Act and the establishment of the General Medical Council.[12] Professionalism is a way of organising and controlling work with an associated ideology of invoking 'partnership' rather than an 'employer—employee' relationship as a basis for negotiation over terms and conditions of providing 'service'. It involves a system of self-government allowing control over entry into the profession through control of education and training, and control not only over the occupation's own work but also the work of others involved in the provision of related services. The pursuit of such control over work is common to many occupations but doctors' and other professions' autonomy is unique in being justified as in the public interest: they and they alone have the knowledge and authority to take decisions on patient care and hence on wider medical issues, and this professional freedom is claimed as essential to good medical care. It is important to distinguish between the historical reasons for the dominance of the medical profession and these arguments used to justify that dominance.

Freidson makes a distinction between autonomy over the *content*, the technological aspects of work, and the *terms*, the social and economic organisation of that work,[13] and suggests that the former is critical to the power of the profession. Such a distinction may be analytically useful but it is clear that the British medical profession, or sectors of it, do not make use of it, as challenges to either are equally resisted. The challenges discussed here are seen by the profession as challenges to both kinds of autonomy, to both clinical and professional freedom. However, as will be shown, the conception of freedom that is being defended is somewhat illusory for many members of the medical profession.

The first challenge considered here is to the existing medical monopoly of knowledge and practice as being of benefit to the public.

The Limits to Medicine: A Change in Priorities?

Ivan Illich has written, 'The medical establishment has become a major threat to health. The disabling impact of professional control over medicine has reached the proportions of an epidemic.'[14] This is perhaps the most extreme formulation of the increasing questioning of the efficiency, effectiveness and even beneficence of much of modern medical care. Freidson suggests that a necessary, though not sufficient, condition of doctors' autonomy is public *belief* in the efficacy of its work.[15] Belief is not necessarily dependent on demonstrable effectiveness but challenges to medical expertise may undermine belief in the legitimacy of medical dominance on the part of patients and health workers, even among doctors themselves.

McKeown has described the history of medicine in Britain as divisible into three stages, up to 1937, 1937 to 1954, and 1954 onwards.[16] It was the first stage that brought the greatest part of all improvements in standards of health, as measured by mortality rates and life expectancy, particularly those of infants. These improvements were achieved not by medical technology as such, but by limiting the spread of infection, by better standards of living and sanitation, and by birth control.[17] During the second stage, further changes in early life disease patterns were brought about by antimicrobial drugs in addition to public health measures. The success of these drugs led to the increasing dominance of a particular theory of disease aetiology, and hence treatment, characterised by McKeown as an 'engineering approach' to medicine.[18] In this approach the body is conceived of as a machine capable of being taken apart and reassembled, 'cured' by active intervention.

The third stage of medicine has seen the increasing dominance of this engineering approach with its dependence on the modern hospital. However, the very success of this approach against infectious diseases has resulted in a major shift in morbidity from those diseases of early life which it can and has cured, to those against which it is relatively powerless; those of degeneration and maladaptation affecting an ageing population. The result has been one of diminishing returns as measured by days lost through sickness, mortality rates and life expectancy in relation to the significant increases in health services expenditure since the inception of the NHS.[19]

In so far as this third stage of medicine coincides more or less with the development of the NHS, it is salutary to point out that the spiralling growth of health expenditure since 1948 is quite opposite to what was forecast under the 'Beveridge illusion', that morbidity, and hence the demand for health care was finite and that once the initial unmet needs of the population were met, expenditure on health care would fall. A second feature of the NHS has been the lack of significant reduction in the different standards of health and health services provision (and the two are by no means to be equated) between different social classes and geographical areas within the NHS.[20]

Cochrane, in a now classic essay,[21] has suggested that many established medical techniques are of dubious and certainly unproven effectiveness. Doctors are trained for the most part in intervention. The dangers of non-treatment and non-diagnosis are seen as greater than the dangers of treatment and over-diagnosis. Negligence is of more concern than iatrogenesis.[22] There is growing concern that heroic procedures cause undue suffering to patients without any tangible benefit and divert scarce resources from other patients. In this sense, one doctor's claim for clinical freedom to treat his individual patients is a restriction on another doctor's ability to help his patients. As David Owen, former Minister of State for Health and himself a doctor, observed, in calling for more cost-consciousness among doctors:

> Clinical freedom is not an abstract concept. Its full realisation demands that the profession faces the practical economic facts of life. The constraints on total resources mean that doctors acting individually can constrain the clinical freedom of their colleagues and also limit the effectiveness of health care for other patients.[23]

McKeown has suggested, given the diminishing returns of curative medicine, and the intractable nature of most major diseases, that the emphasis in medicine should shift from 'cure' to care. Any change in emphasis in medicine implies changes in the allocation of resources. Control over the allocation of resources in health care is, as the comments by David Owen indicate, seen as an essential part of clinical freedom by individual doctors. Attempts to reallocate resources are often resisted on the grounds that they limit (the losing doctor's) clinical freedom.

The question of inappropriate allocation of resources, especially prominent in the financial crisis of the time, was taken up in the 'Priorities Document' produced in the spring of 1976.[24] This recommended that the limited expansion proposed in current expenditure on the health services up to 1979/80 be concentrated on primary care (3.8 per cent growth per year) and on services for the growing number of elderly people (3.2 per cent growth per year), the mentally handicapped (2.8 per cent), and the mentally ill (1.8 per cent). Acute hospital services would get a proportionately smaller increase of 1.2 per cent per annum and maternity services an actual cut in their allocation of 1.8 per cent, on the grounds of the falling birth rate. The intention here is not to discuss the merits of the proposals but the profession's reaction to them. Their reaction illustrates how the allocation of resources in the NHS to date has been determined by the relative power of different groups within the medical profession and of the profession as against other groups, and attempts to change this distribution are resisted by those who stand to lose.

Thus the document was greeted by a *British Medical Journal* leader writer as: 'a policy of despair, and it reflects the Department's refusal over the years to recognise the really fundamental issues that must be resolved if the NHS is to survive as a first-class health service.'[25] Apart from begging the question as to what the fundamental issues are, and who is responsible for determining them, the leader does not recognise any of the 'diminishing returns' arguments identified above. The claim is made that in the long run money spent on medical research and the acute hospital sector (and it is assumed the two are identical) will lead to improvement in the treatment of the 'really common diseases' of today such as coronary thrombosis. The thrust of arguments like those of Powles [26] and others is that this has not been so in the past. Recognition of this (as well as cost-reduction) is one factor behind the 'priorities' proposals.

The leader condemns proposals to cut maternity services' resources on the grounds that this will not help the efforts to reduce perinatal mortality which in turn will reduce the number of surviving handicapped children.[27] There is no apparent concern for the conditions under which the existing handicapped are cared for. Rather than any change in the allocation of resources to the profession, the leader recommends a sustained health education programme aimed at prevention. (This may appear to involve a change in resource allocation but the present and proposed health education budget represents less than 1 per cent of current health service expenditure per annum.)

The inability of non-professionals to assess priorities is made clear by the leader writer: 'By putting "people before buildings" and by giving practical expression to public sympathy for the old and the handicapped Mrs. Castle has, perhaps, allowed sentiment to over-rule intellect.'[28] This view would not appear to be shared by Sir George Godber, former Chief Medical Officer at the DHSS, who wrote that 'Buildings, of course, are not the main factors in the quality of hospital care. Good staff can do good work in a barn.'[29] While this leader is most unlikely to represent the views of the entire profession, it is an illustration of the vehement negative response to proposals for change that the medical profession's leaders have displayed in the past.[30] Yet a close reading of the proposals shows that the threats to clinical freedom or the scale of reallocation are not overtly such as to warrant this response. No specific manpower directives are proposed and the absolute lack of such an intention in the case of general practice is quite explicit: 'In general, it is not proposed to intervene in the natural development of the primary care services, as determined by demand and the *professional response* to it.'[31] Nor are any attempts to interfere with individuals' clinical autonomy proposed, though there is an Appendix on 'Innovations in Clinical Practice' as an encouragement to consider cost-effective treatments.

The objections stem from the implications posed for the established structure of the medical profession by a change in priorities away from the acute and maternity hospital sectors to fields where the primacy of the medical profession's role is open to question. These acute and maternity sectors together were estimated in the Priorities Document to have accounted for 43.1 per cent of current and capital NHS expenditure, almost £2,000 millions. Doctors in these sectors are the most powerful and prestigious in the profession. Through, for example, the oldest Royal Colleges (Physicians, Surgeons, Obstetricians and Gynaecologists) they have been dominant in decision-making and resource allocation in medicine.[32] This position has been reflected at least in the past by their prominence in medical school curricula and subsequently in students' career choice,[33] and in the distribution of Merit or Distinction Awards. Distinction Awards are special payments awarded to consultants for distinguished contributions to medicine, not for services to the NHS. This was made clear by the consultants' leaders' response to proposals made in December 1974 to replace them in their present form with some form of long-service award. Great secrecy surrounds decisions over their allocation, which is largely in the profession's hands at national level through a committee currently chaired by the President of the Royal College of Obstetricians and Gynaecologists. Concern has often been expressed that they are distributed in favour of the high-technology acute specialities, as against the lower-prestige, less competitive geriatrics and psychiatry, etc.

The third stage of medicine has brought about a proliferation of new medical specialities and sub-specialities.[34] These may be dichotomised roughly into those which have developed from technological advances in acute medical and surgical treatment such as thoracic surgery and neuro-surgery, and those which have developed in response to the changing morbidity patterns of an ageing society, notably geriatrics, rheumatology and rehabilitation. The former tend to show a better than average distribution of Distinction Awards and the latter worse, showing that youth is not a sufficient explanation of the uneven distribution of awards. In 1974, 33.9 per cent of all consultants held a Merit Award; 73 per cent of thoracic surgeons and 63.4 per cent of neuro-surgeons held one as compared with 23 per cent of geriatricians.[35] The uneven distribution is sometimes defended on the grounds that it is easier to measure 'excellence' in the acute specialities, but, as the discussion on the diminishing returns of these specialities suggests, this begs the question of the criteria by which 'excellence' might be measured and by whom.

Divisions between specialities within medicine are one case of divisions within the profession which will be returned to below. They are discussed here to illustrate the way that proposals for changes in the organisation of medical care challenge the dominance and hence the autonomy of certain sectors of the medical profession. They also pose questions as to the legitimacy of medical dominance over other health workers and over patients.

Dominance and the Division of Labour: Changes in Relationships with Other Health Workers

If doctors' techniques are ineffective there is no justification for their dominance in the medical division of labour either at the workplace or in policy-making. This would be the logical consequence of accepting some of the arguments of writers such as Powles, Cochrane and Illich. Doctors' autonomy is justified on the grounds of their monopoly of knowledge and effective techniques. This justification is of a different order to the historical reasons for medical dominance over other health workers. The historical explanation must include their effective organisation and their dominant class and sex position relative to other groups. Studies by Johnson and the Parrys suggest that the gaining of occupational control in the form of 'professionalism' is only likely where 'an occupational group shares, by virtue of its membership of a dominant class or caste, wider resources of power. . .'[36] Developments both within medicine and in society as a whole, such as the greater political strength of trade unions, have led to increasing challenges to medical dominance by other health workers.

Developments in medical technology and changes in morbidity have led to a proliferation of new branches of medicine and health-related occupations. The emphasis on hospital medicine since the establishment of the NHS in particular has resulted in massive increases in the labour force.[37] The delivery of health services in hospital and increasingly in general practice is a highly complex affair involving not merely those who provide direct services for patients—nurses, therapists, doctors and some technical staff—but also the clerical and administrative staff and ancillary workers necessary for running large residential organisations.

Even in those fields where the scope for specifically medical intervention may be limited, patient care remains formally under medical control.[38] Consultants have had control of the nursing, paramedical and technical services and have tended to regard the administrative machinery as a means of achieving their own ends.[39] In general practice, the development of primary care as a speciality concerned with the 'whole patient' in his social environment, and the changing standards of practice, has involved the doctor in closer association with health

visitors, community nurses and social workers and clerical and recep-
tion staff. With the exception of social workers, these groups are
medically controlled. Social workers have resisted incorporation into
the medical arena and this has been formally recognised in the 1974
reorganisation's separation of health and personal social services.

Developments in modern medicine have perhaps sown the seeds of
destruction for medical dominance in its traditional form. Not only
have they led to the possible limits of doctors' efficacy and hence undermined the legitimacy of dominance, but they have provided the
possibility of other occupations developing their own occupational
strategies and organisation, either through professionalism or unionism.
The state's role has been critical in altering conditions affecting occupational strength both at the workplace and at the national level largely
as a result of pressure for centralisation and administrative efficiency.[40]
The 1974 reorganisation is an example of how these pressures in
shaping the new structure have (unintentionally) reinforced the growing
tendency for staff as opposed to medical or administrative control. This
can be illustrated by an increasingly recognised role in decision-making
and management given the nursing profession, reflecting a changing
status relative to doctors. Nursing officers are members of management
teams at all tiers in the reorganised service even though at the level of
patient care the role of the nurse has changed little.

A more recent dramatic challenge to medical autonomy has come
not from those whose skills are more appropriate for a caring approach
to health care but from those whose role in medical care is very much
linked to the large modern hospital, the ancillary workers. Dimmock
has described how the belief that labour relations in the health services
were qualitatively different from those in industry was shaken by the
1973 Ancillaries' Dispute. The moral embargo on strikes against the
patients' interests was broken and, more significantly, ancillary workers
became involved in decision-making at the local level in what had hitherto been seen as medical matters, not least in the question of what
constitutes an emergency.[41] The ancillary workers justified their actions
as being *for the benefit of patients,* that better pay and conditions
would help to alleviate staff shortages and thereby improve patient care.
Patients' welfare is an argument that can and has been used by any group
of health workers: by ancillary workers and junior doctors to justify
strike action; by the Health Service unions to justify their campaign for
phasing out 'paybeds' from the NHS; and by their opponents in favour
of private practice; and by politicians to justify all their actions. As Ham
has pointed out, patients as a group are the least able to present their

arguments.[42]

The experience of the 1973 and subsequent disputes and the realisation of their ability to disrupt services was an important factor in the pre-emptive moves at Charing Cross Hospital in 1974 by NUPE members opposed to private medicine. These moves were a direct challenge to consultants' power. The action was condemned in both the national and medical press as undemocratic, with the view expressed that 'Parliament, not the unions, must decide.'[43] However, when, as a result of this altered balance of power, the phasing out of private facilities became a central part of Labour Party policy, and the possibility of Parliament 'deciding' began to look like a reality, then the issue was recast and the medical press claimed infringements of clinical freedom. The strength of the Health Service unions enabled or indeed pressurised the Labour government elected in 1974 to take action on an issue that had been in the background since 1948 when Bevan 'failed' (in his view[44] and that of the left) to separate private and NHS facilities because of consultant opposition. That the issue was revived in the seventies is an indication of the increasing strength of groups other than doctors. That the Bill submitted to Parliament is a considerable modification of the union's original proposals is an indication that the profession's ability to influence decisions is still very strong.

Doctors' ability to influence decisions rests in part in the sanction they can theoretically exercise, withdrawal of services. Significantly, militant action in the form of working to contract and strike threats has only recently become a tactic used by doctors, following the example of the ancillary workers and radiographers. In January 1975, following the breakdown of the Owen Working Party on private practice and consultants' contracts, and the rejection of a backdated pay demand,[45] many consultants started working to rule. Junior doctors have threatened strike action over the implementation of their new contracts during 1975 and 1976. These actions contrast markedly with the traditional form of protest favoured by the British Medical Association, to call for resignations from the Health Service. As a sanction it has never been shown to be seen as a realistic possibility by the majority of its members. In January 1976 a ballot was held of all consultants over the 'Goodman proposals' to phase out paybeds.[46] The alternative to acceptance of the proposals was resignation from the service as the 'ultimate weapon in industrial action'. Only 54 per cent of consultants voted and of these only 20 per cent voted for resignation.[47] The use of more militant tactics by doctors, or rather by some doctors, points up the need to analyse changes within the profession and in the relationship between the leaders of the profession and the majority of its members, in accounting for the current dissatisfaction among doctors.

Changes and Divisions within the Profession

For simplicity, 'the medical profession' has frequently been referred to in this paper as if it were a uniform body with a common response to challenges and changes and with all its members enjoying a common degree of autonomy. The discussion of the Priorities Document and Distinction Awards indicated this was not so. Divisions and differences within the profession have always had a profound effect on the shape of the health services [48] and these divisions and the relations between them are not constant over time. The medical profession is best described, like most occupational groups, as 'loose amalgamations of segments pursuing different objectives in different manners and more or less delicately held together under a common name at a particular period of history'.[49]

The origins and form of these divisions are often not explicable in terms of medicine alone, but stem from the wider social context in which medicine and the medical profession exist. The structure of the health labour force as a whole in Britain (and also the USA) is a microcosm of the labour force as a whole in terms of its stratification by social class, sex and race.[50] The latter two dimensions of stratification have become increasingly salient within the medical profession. Medicine developed during the second half of the nineteenth century as a predominantly white male middle-class profession. The second half of the twentieth century has seen something of a change. In 1975 approximately one-fifth of all practising doctors in the NHS were women and one-third overseas-born.[51] That women and overseas doctors are disproportionately employed in the low-status specialities discussed earlier and in low-grade posts both reflects and reinforces their low status. In 1975, 85 per cent of registrars in geriatrics were overseas-born compared with 40 per cent in general medicine. The equivalent percentages at consultant level were 34 and 9.4 per cent respectively. Women represent more than 50 per cent of doctors employed in the community health services, but are mostly at the clinical medical officer level, rather than holding the con-sultant-level posts as specialists in community medicine.

Concern is frequently expressed that the UK is too dependent on overseas doctors and that, as this source of supply is showing signs of drying up, expansion of home medical school output is necessary.[52] Women doctors are also seen as a problem because, so the argument runs, they form an increasing proportion of qualifying doctors but, through insufficient use of their skills, do not show an adequate return on society's investment. It is not the intention here to analyse the validity of these arguments in detail though the problems of hospital staffing will be taken up later.[53] That these two categories are seen as 'problems' illustrates their lack of representation in decision-making on medical manpower policy. There is an increasing distinction between junior posts that are part of an organised training scheme and those that are primarily service posts[54] and these minority doctors are over-represented in the latter. The medical labour market can be seen as a special case of the 'dual labour market' found in other spheres.[55] This concept suggests that labour markets can often be divided into primary and secondary sectors along dimensions such as pay, recruitment and turnover. Primary sector posts are ordered into hierarchical sets with recruitment to higher posts predominantly from within these sets. Thus, vocational training schemes with rotating registrar posts represent primary sector posts. The secondary sector in contrast is not internally structured; recruits come from outside the organisation and leave on completion of a specific job without promotion. This stratification of posts is linked to the stratification of holders of posts by, for example, race and sex. Over time, these two dimensions of stratification become conflated and a vicious circle set up. Low-status, poorly paid posts tend to be women's posts and vice versa. In the NHS, the situation is represented by women doctors who take on part-time posts or clinical assistantships not recognised for training purposes, and by the overseas doctors who are only granted temporary registration linked to a specific post.

The concern over the possible ending of the supply of overseas doctors has re-focused attention on the position of junior hospital doctors as a whole, and their dissatisfactions. Junior doctors, simultaneously providing service and undergoing training, and dissatisfied with their pay and conditions, have been a feature of hospital life since the early nineteenth century when they *paid for* the privilege of doing the basic hospital work while learning from the (honorary) consultants. This structure was formalised under the NHS with the provision of a larger and more secure income for both groups of doctors.[56] However, hours and conditions of service and above all career prospects in terms of getting consultant posts have not improved to the same extent. Part of the junior doctors' dissatisfaction stems from promotion 'delayed by the staffing structure of the hospitals rather than by their own stage of fitness for responsibility'.[57] This raises the question to be developed later of how and by whom medical staffing is determined.

The increasing demand for labour associated with the modern hospital has affected doctors as much as other health workers with most of the increase being in the junior categories who provide routine patient care. Between 1937 and 1947, the number of non-consultant posts is estimated to have risen from 2,400 to 8,200 whereas the number of consultant posts rose only from 3,000 to about 4,000.[58] Under the NHS this trend has continued. Between 1956 and 1974, the number of doctors in junior training grades rose from 8,071 to 19,762 (140 per cent), far greater than the increased output from medical schools, and the number of consultant posts from 6,490 to 11,459 (70 per cent).[59] Analysis of the expansion of hospital posts by grade since 1948 shows a move down the 'ladder' which reflects the outcome of the interaction of the three parties with interests in hospital staffing structures; the state concerned to staff hospitals at minimum cost; the medical establishment anxious to preserve remuneration, etc. for its members and to prevent dilution of their autonomy; and the local health administration who have to provide patient care.[60]

Junior doctors have until very recently been absent from negotiations regarding staffing structures and hence their career prospects. Thus, despite the formal objective in the last four years of preferential growth of consultant rather than junior posts, no such growth has been achieved. Between 1974 and 1975, the number of consultant posts increased by 2.5 per cent but the increase in junior posts was almost 8 per cent.[61] Consultant expansion in particular, though often proposed,[62] has been resisted by the state on cost grounds and on occasions by the medical establishment, whether at national policy or at local level, on the grounds that it might lead to lowering of standards and, by implication, loss of autonomy and even remuneration. At the same time, they have often defended the pyramidal structure of hospital staffing. They have opposed both attempts to restrict the expansion of junior grades and any attempts to relieve the resultant bottleneck either by expansion of consultant posts or a non-consultant grade, as in the case of the redundant registrars of the 1950s.[63]

In many specialties within hospital medicine, the situation facing junior doctors is similar to that of the fifties. Career prospects have perhaps worsened; not only are there no more consultant posts, but the alternatives in general practice for those who 'fall off the ladder', envisaged by the Spens Committee in recommending this competitive apprenticeship system, are not as open as they were then. The rise in the status of general practice has made entry more competitive and the proposed introduction of mandatory vocational training for principals may exclude doctors who have not made it an early career choice. A second alternative for the dissatisfied or unemployed doctor is emigration. There is little accurate information on current levels of emigration (one recent estimate suggested 600 per annum with no indication of sources).[64] The interpretation of statistics on emigration is highly problematic[65] but it is clear that despite the establishment of free movement of doctors within the EEC, many of the developed countries, particularly the USA, share the same problems of an over-supply of doctors in some fields and locations, and an acute shortage in the unattractive ones. Emigration is increasingly only possible to 'unattractive posts'.

There is now a situation in which many junior doctors are unable to find satisfactory career posts. Yet, medical schools are the only sector of higher education undergoing expansion, in order to lessen dependence on foreign doctors. The Todd Report recommended increases in student intake leading to an output of 3,500 graduates in 1975-9 and 4,250 in 1985-9. These figures have subsequently been revised upwards, and are unlikely to be met; they would in any case not meet for some time the estimate of 4,500 doctors needed annually to replace the overseas doctors. The number of doctors needed annually to replace consultants and general practitioners who retire or die each year is estimated as only 2,500.[66] The target of 4,500 new doctors is derived from a situation in which there is a large turnover of overseas doctors every year. Home-produced graduates are unlikely to behave in the same manner and the demand for new recruits could be considerably less. (The assumption that the number of incoming doctors will fall permanently is open to question unless there is further legislation.)[67] Unless there is a major expansion in consultant posts or restructuring in hospital staffing, which seems unlikely in the light of current attitudes towards public expenditure, it is difficult to see where many of these newly trained doctors are going to find permanent career posts when they have completed their 'training'.

Junior doctors have lacked autonomy both in hospitals, where they are responsible to consultants for their clinical work, and at the national level in determining the terms of their work, for they have not been a party to negotiations between government and their seniors, whose interests may not be the same as theirs. While service provision is formally in the hands of the state, medical education and training, and therefore the supply of junior doctors, is largely in the profession's hands. Educational policies can and have been manipulated to solve staffing problems without radical reform; the acute problems of staffing casualty departments in the fifties was slightly relieved by the introduction of a period of casualty service as a requirement for the

Fellowship of the Royal College of Surgeons.[68] Such adjustments have not always been in the interests of junior doctors.[69]

The very growth in numbers that has led to this dissatisfaction among junior doctors has also been an influence on the strategy eventually adopted by them. The same factors leading to a more militant and organised industrial relations stance among nurses, radiographers and ancillary workers have affected junior doctors. They have in the past been dependent on the consultants whose jobs they hope to inherit. As this prospect diminishes, so alternative strategies are adopted. By perceiving that they have not always benefited from the 'partnership' that professional autonomy involves between the state and the doctors' leaders, junior doctors have attempted to enter into direct negotiation on employer–employee lines and have negotiated a contract which specifies the number of hours to be worked and incorporates payment for overtime.[70] That such a contract is a significant departure from the ideology of professionalism was noted by the Independent Review Body who somewhat grudgingly accepted their claims.[71] The adoption of the principle of overtime payments together with the terms of the Social Contract which allows overtime payments but prevents salary increments over £8,500 have significantly reduced the financial advantages of promotion from senior registrar to consultant. While this may be only a temporary feature, it does indicate the significant gains made by junior doctors during the last three years by pursuing policies of their own rather than relying on those whose autonomy they hope to inherit.

The organised strength of junior doctors has had an impact on the established leadership of the profession in the form of the BMA. Challenges to the BMA, which has often been regarded as primarily representing the general practitioners, are not new but the level of growth of two particular alternative organisations is unprecedented. These are the Junior Hospital Doctors' Association[72] and the Hospital Consultants and Specialists' Association,[73] which in the summer of 1976 united as the British Hospital Doctors' Federation to pursue their common aims more effectively.

At present, the BMA still has a formal monopoly over negotiations with the DHSS, applications for negotiating rights for both the JHDA and HCSA having been rejected. This suggests that there are possible advantages perceived by the state in maintaining their existing relationship with the BMA. The HCSA applied unsuccessfully to the Industrial Relations Court in 1974 for negotiating rights. Rather than concede, the BMA in turn attempted to negotiate integration with the HCSA. The JHDA strength outside the BMA was an important factor in the granting of autonomous status to the Hospital Junior Staffs Group Council, now the Hospital Junior Staffs Committee. In 1972, Sir Paul Chambers produced his proposals for streamlining the the BMA's rather cumbersome structure,[74] partly in response to new industrial relations legislation and partly in response to the forthcoming reorganisation. However, the Chambers' proposals appeared to involve a reduction in the autonomy of the different craft committees and a reduction in peripheral representation, i.e. the very areas in which the BMA faced challenges.[75] The proposals were eventually rejected after long debate and the final shape of the new constitution showed very clearly the divisions within the profession and the concern on the part of the BMA's leadership that if all interests, particularly those of juniors, were not adequately represented within the BMA, doctors would go elsewhere.[76]

It is in this context that during 1976 two particularly interesting issues have been raised in the pages of the BMJ; first the possible desirability of a closed shop on the grounds that many doctors are benefiting from the BMA's services without paying for them; and, secondly, even more antithetical to the ideology of professionalism, the possibility of TUC affiliation has been raised. That these possibilities even find their way on to the pages of a professional journal may well be signalling the beginnings of fundamental changes in the way the profession looks at itself, its relations with government and its role in society.

Discussion of the structure of the BMA and its ability to represent the different professional interests has usually been in terms of the 'tri-partite division' of medicine into general practice, hospital and community (formerly local authority) medicine.[77] The discussion above suggests that *divisions within* the hospital category may be growing in importance. What of the present relations between the three major categories?

The most heralded feature of the 1974 reorganisation has been the unification of the tripartite administrative structure. Since the Porritt Report[78] issued by the physicians in 1962, the principle of unification of the Service had been widely accepted as desirable among doctors but there was little agreement as to what form the unified Service might take.

Analysis of the response to successive proposals for reorganisation shows that each group responded in terms of its own concerns, preferring, and for the most part gaining, a structure that was most similar to that currently experienced. Thus, throughout the period of negotiation, i.e. from the first Green Paper[79] in 1968 up to 1 April 1974, general practitioners were concerned to retain their independent contractor status, and succeeded with the creation of Family Practitioner

Committees to replace Local Executive Councils. Hospital consultants were concerned to have continued access to decision-making. This concern was expressed, for example, in response to the second Green Paper,[80] when it was argued that the areas proposed were simultaneously too large and remote from the individual hospital and too small because they involved fragmentation of the existing regional hospital boards.[81] Hospital and general practice doctors were united only in their opposition to greater centralisation and to local authority control. The group most affected by reorganisation in so far as they faced leaving local authority employment for the Health Service appeared to have most favoured health areas with boundaries coterminous with local authorities. In so far as there was no unification in the mode of employment, the resultant structure of the Service as far as doctors are concerned is better described as 'partial co-ordination' rather than as integration.[82]

In contrast to the furore that accompanied negotiations leading up to the Appointed Day in 1948, the discussion prior to the 1974 re-organisation took place with relatively little interest or involvement by the vast majority of clinicians. This was partly because the re-organisation was seen as merely a matter of administrative reform not affecting the structure of the profession, and probably partly because the plethora of complex proposals was confusing to a profession that during the period of discussion was concerned with more immediate issues, notably with pay, with the debate over the future of the General Medical Council[83] and, latterly, with the question of private practice. Brown and his colleagues, in a study of the reorganised service in Humberside after one year, found that many consultants were ignorant of the workings of the advisory machinery their leaders had negotiated for them.[84] He points out that the medical profession's involvement in re-organisation discussions was predominantly at the national level 'where they took the lead...but on the local stage the roles were reversed...the clinicians played [no] more than a minor part in applying the structure to local conditions'.[85] This gap between the leaders of the profession (intent on obtaining maximal involvement in decision-making for doctors without regard for the time commitments involved) and the clinicians who were then called upon to operate the resultant advisory and decision-making machinery, reflects in part the profession's orientation to its partnership with the state rather than to the workplace. It is an important factor in the discontent with reorganisation, often expressed in terms of criticisms of administrators, that the Humberside study found.

To a large extent the structure of the re-organised NHS was

> modelled to the desires of the medical profession. . . but having got
> it, the doctors did not seem particularly satisfied. . . having sought
> and obtained a role in management, it was clear that many doctors
> did not know what to do with it.[86]

As Brown has indicated, the final structure was modelled not so much
to the desires of *the* medical profession but to the differing desires of
different sectors, or rather of the leaders of different sectors. For example, the management arrangements set out in the 'Grey Book'[87] bore
'distinct marks of the profession's influence on the discussions'[88] but
such an influence was not a united one. The eventual composition of
the District Management Team and the concept of consensus management stem from the divisions within the profession. In particular,
opposition to having the community physician as the sole medical
representative on the team led to the situation where there are two
elected and temporary doctor members, responsible to their colleagues,
and one permanent member accountable to the Area Health Authority,
the District Community Physician.[89]

The decision-making and advisory machinery established by reorganisation calls for consensus between a number of different groups which
may be difficult to achieve within medicine as we have seen, apart from
with other groups. We have seen that there may be competition between
speciality groups within hospitals for scarce resources and the establishment of Cogwheel divisions[90] prior to reorganisation did not eliminate
this problem and nor did the new structure, at least as revealed by
Brown's study.

Complaints about the reorganised structure are often focused on the
administration. It is indeed true that by taking decision-making away
from the level of individual hospitals, reorganisation has lessened the
day-to-day contact between consultants and those administrators who
can take decisions. However, the tendency to blame administrators both
at the workplace and at the national level is more widespread. Green,
in a study of three Scottish hospitals, found that conflict between medical staff and the administration was much less significant than conflict
between different groups of professionals. However, the administrators
were usually blamed.

> In making demands for equipment consultants seemed to think
> that if they did not get what they wanted it was the fault of the
> administration. They failed to appreciate, through ignorance or
> choice, that if one specialty did not have its request accepted this

was because other specialties had succeeded.[91]

As shown earlier, some specialities in the past at least have been more powerful than others and attempts to reallocate resources have been largely ineffective because of these sectors' defence of their clinical freedom. Reorganisation was conceived largely in management terms, with the hope that decision-making would be based on consensus as a result of objective informed discussion, rather than recognising the essentially political nature of decisions about allocation of resources.[92] The pursuit of such consensus, to supersede victories for the powerful, seems chimerical, especially if a change in medical priorities is involved. Critics of the profession refer to the need to reduce medical dominance and autonomy, but it is clear that there are sectors of the profession who enjoy little autonomy.

Conclusion

The paper has suggested that the established medical profession faces challenges to its dominant position on several fronts. These challenges affect the doctor both as politician and practitioner. Changes in morbidity render the prevailing medical mode and its associated allocation of priorities increasingly inappropriate. A change in allocation of priorities involves a loss in resources to those who have been able to determine what the priorities should be in the past. A shift from a curative approach to one of care and prevention involves more responsibility and involvement on the part of patients[93] and a greater participation by other health workers. To be powerless in the treatment (or any other) situation is not a condition for which many doctors are trained and may involve considerable personal readjustment.

A second challenge from the other health workers is their increasing organisation, largely through trade unions, and as a result of reorganisation, which is altering the position of doctors in national and local decision-making. They are no longer the sole 'partners' in decision-making, as is recognised, for example, by the proposals for other health workers' representation on health authorities.[94]

Within the profession itself there are changes such that the unity of the profession and the position of the established leadership appears precarious. Critics of the profession have often condemned the syndicalist power of the profession. A less simplistic view of the situation would acknowledge that some sectors of the profession have had very little power *vis-à-vis* their professional 'colleagues'. Autonomy is not evenly distributed through the profession.

The manpower policies of the NHS have been largely of the profession's making through their control over supply (with state support where money-saving was likely). The paradox of this professional autonomy is that what is in the interests of one section of a divided profession may not be in the interests of another. The leaders of the profession have enjoyed partnership with the state, not shared by their junior colleagues. Because financial and formal or ultimate responsibility for the service rests with the state, the profession's spokesmen have repeatedly been able to lay the blame for faults in the service on 'the NHS', from which they often exclude themselves. They have excused themselves from taking responsibility for faults which may be in part of their own making on the grounds that they deliver on their side of the bargain, and only they can judge how well they do that.

> At every stage the doctors have judged their 'partner', the state, by the extent to which it is willing to fund the service adequately— on their definition of adequacy—and maintain appropriate levels of remuneration—on their definition of appropriate.[95]

The profession's response to these challenges has been in terms of a defence of their autonomy in the public interest. For example, 'Patients before Politics' is the slogan of the Campaign for Independence in Medicine, a pressure group opposed to the Labour government's proposals to separate private medicine from NHS hospitals. As we have seen, if 'Patients before Politics' means putting the patients' interests before political dogma then this is a claim that can and has been made by both sides, depending in part on which patients are being considered. If it is taken as an expression of the possibility or even desirability for taking 'politics out of medicine', then this is unrealistic in implying that judgements about where priorities in health care should lie are neutral clinical questions. Nor would it be in the interests of the profession as a whole in so far as the eminent position of the medical profession today has been brought about by political activity, not solely by attending to the interests of patients.

Aneurin Bevan wrote in his autobiography: 'to speak of the medical profession is not the same as to speak of the individuals in it', and his hardest task was 'overcoming the fears, real and imaginary, of the medical profession'.[96] The intention of this paper is to begin to identify the real issues facing the medical profession.

The defence of 'autonomy' by any occupational group is understandable in the face of challenge. It is not necessarily in the interests of all members of the profession, the Health Service as a whole, or patients. The ultimate problem for the Health Service, in which doctors play a central part, is how, through politics, patient interests may be best served.

Notes

1. For a recent study of the ways by which this position was achieved see N. Parry and J. Parry, *The Rise of the Medical Profession,* Croom Helm, London, 1975.
2. The paper concentrates on clinicians and if the emphasis is on hospital doctors this is because most of the recent changes discussed have affected hospital doctors, as opposed to general practitioners, to a far greater extent. This is in marked contrast to the situation up to ten years or even five years ago when it was the general practitioners who saw their prospects as threatened. See M. Jefferys, 'The Doctor's Dilemma—A Sociological Viewpoint', *Social and Economic Administration,* 4, 1970.
3. E. Friedson, *Professional Dominance,* Atherton, New York, 1970, p.154.
4. See Parry and Parry, op. cit., and also D. G. Gill, 'The British National Health Service: professional determinants of administrative structure', *International Journal of Health Services,* 1, 4, 1971, pp.347-53.
5. *British Medical Journal Supplement,* 1 May 1976, p.1086. Parallel to the situation thirty years ago, the Health Service Bill proposals can be seen as increasing the independence of those members of the profession who benefit from existing private medicine facilities by guaranteeing its continued existence. See, for example, *On Call,* 17 August 1976, pp.8-9. That the Bill is based on the 'Goodman proposals' with an independent board overseeing the phasing out is an indication of the considerable strength of the profession rather than of weakness.
6. See, for example, R. Stevens, *Medical Practice in Modern England,* Yale University Press, New Haven, 1966, and G. Forsyth, *Doctors and State Medicine,* Pitman Medical, London, 1966.
7. The challenge from patients is considered elsewhere in this volume—see Ham and Johnson.
8. Parry and Parry, op. cit., p.212, and Stevens, op. cit., pp.259-69.
9. The classic study of the relationships between the government and the medical profession as represented by the BMA between 1946 and 1958 remains H. Eckstein, *Pressure Group Politics,* Allen and Unwin, London, 1960.
10. E. Freidson, *Profession of Medicine,* Dodd Mead, New York, 1972, p.23.
11. See, for example, J. B. McKinlay, 'On the Professional Regulation of Change' in P. Halmos (ed.), *Professionalisation and Social Change,* Sociological Review Monograph No 20. 1973, pp.61-84, and T. J. Johnson, *Professions and Power,* Macmillan, London, 1972.
12. Parry and Parry, op. cit., and also, 'The Teacher and Professionalism: the Failure of an Occupational Strategy' in M. Flude and J. Ahier, *Educability, Schools and Ideology,* Croom Helm, London, 1974, pp.160-85.
13. Freidson, op. cit., 1970, p.84.
14. I. Illich, *Limits to Medicine,* Marion Boyars, London, 1976, p.3.
15. Freidson, op. cit., 1970, p.12.
16. T. McKeown, 'A Sociological Approach to the History of Medicine' in G. McLachlan and T. McKeown (eds.), *Medical History and Medical Care,* Nuffield Provincial Hospitals Trust, Oxford, 1971, pp.1-16.

17. As Powles has pointed out, birth control was vigorously opposed by the established medical profession in the nineteenth century. J. Powles, 'On the Limitations of Modern Medicine', *Social Science and Man*, 1, 1973, pp.1-30.

18. McKeown, 'A Historical Appraisal of the Medical Task', in McLachlan and McKeown (eds.), op. cit., p.36.

19. See Powles, op. cit., and P. Draper, G. Best and T. Dennis, *Health, Money and the National Health Service*, Unit for the Study of Health Policy, Department of Community Medicine, Guy's Hospital Medical School, London, 1976.

20. P. Townsend, 'Inequality and the Health Service', *The Lancet*, 15 June 1974, pp.1179-90.

21. A. L. Cochrane, *Effectiveness and Efficiency: Random Reflections on Health Services*, Nuffield Provincial Hospitals Trust, London, 1972.

22. In the United States this is clearly so as the spiralling rate of malpractice suits, predominantly for negligence, may result in doctors practising 'defensive medicine'. See N. Hershey, 'The Defensive Practice of Medicine, Myth or Reality?', *Milbank Memorial Fund Quarterly*, 1972.

23. D. Owen, 'Clinical Freedom and Professional Freedom', *The Lancet*, 8 May 1976, p.1008.

24. Separate and different consultative documents were produced for England, Wales and Scotland. All references here are to the English one—Department of Health and Social Security, *Priorities for Health and Social Services in England: A Consultative Document*, HMSO, London, April 1976.

25. *British Medical Journal*, 3 April 1976, p.788.

26. Powles, op. cit., pp.12-13 on the ineffectiveness of intensive coronary care.

27. This claim and others made in this leader, and in a second one—*British Medical Journal*, 12 June 1976, pp.1425-6—were heavily criticised in subsequent correspondence, e.g. *British Medical Journal*, 24 April 1976, pp.1013-14.

28. *British Medical Journal*, 3 April 1976, p.787.

29. G. Godber, *The Health Service, Past, Present and Future*, Athlone Press, University of London, 1975, p.27.

30. See A. Bevan, *In Place of Fear*, MacGibbon and Kee, London, 1961, p.110.

31. DHSS, *Priorities for Health*, op. cit., p.17 (emphasis added).

32. See Stevens, op. cit.

33. *Royal Commission on Medical Education 1961-68* (Todd Report), HMSO, London, 1968, Appendix 19.

34. Stevens, op. cit., pp.336-52; Godber, op. cit., p.28.

35. P. Bruggen and S. Bourne, 'Further Examination of the Distinction Awards System in England and Wales', *British Medical Journal*, 28 February 1976, pp.536-7. They also point out that of community physicians given consultant status as a result of the 1974 reorganisation, only 16 (2.9 per cent) had been granted an award. See Towell, this volume, for a fuller discussion of the status of the community physician *vis-à-vis* his clinical colleagues.

36. Johnson, op. cit., p.43 and Parry and Parry, op. cit.

37. See Dimmock, this volume.

38. Critics of the medical profession have suggested that the development of some specialities is an attempt to maintain (inappropriate) medical dominance. Whatever the reason, the organisation of patient care is structured around the consultant or the general practitioner. For example, in the case of the mentally handicapped, there may be little role for a doctor but 'patients' remain under medical control. In a residential unit for the mentally handicapped recently brought to the author's attention, overall responsibility for patient care was in the hands of a geriatrician.

39. C. Davies, 'Professionals in organisations: Some preliminary observations of

hospital consultants', *Sociological Review,* 4, 20, 1972, pp.553-67.
40. See Dimmock, this volume.
41. See R. F. Dyson, *The Ancillary Staff Industrial Action: Spring, 1973,* Leeds Regional Hospital Board, Leeds, 1974.
42. See Ham, this volume.
43. *On Call,* 8 July 1974, p.8.
44. Bevan, op. cit., p. 115.
45. The Owen Working Party of Consultants and the DHSS was set up in June 1974 by the newly elected Labour government to look at the related questions of consultants' contracts and the paybed issue. The two sides proved deadlocked and the final breakdown was precipitated by the publication in November 1974 of proposals for what appeared to the doctors' representatives to be a full-time salaried service with 'full commitment allowances' as incentives to participate. There was also a timetable for the phasing out of paybeds from NHS hospitals. Consultants in the North-east started working to rule almost immediately and in January 1975, rather than lose support, the BMA officially sanctioned the action. Aggravating the situation was the simultaneous dispute over an 18 per cent demand backdated to April 1974 which was rejected by the Independent Review Body on Doctors and Dentists' Pay, not because it was not deserved, but because it contravened the Social Contract. The independence of the Review Body was challenged and the Chairman, Lord Halsbury, resigned.
46. See note 5.
47. *British Medical Journal Supplement,* 1 May 1976, p.1087. The lack of strike action among British doctors, as among other health workers, has fostered the illusion of its impossibility. Doctors in other countries, notably Belgium, Italy, Canada and Chile, have adopted strike action over a variety of issues— see R. Belmar and V. W. Sidel, 'An International Perspective on Strikes and Strike Threats of Physicians: the case of Chile', *Int. J. Health Services,* 5, 1, 1975, pp.53-64.
48. Gill, op. cit., 1971.
49. R. Bucher and A. Strauss, 'Professions in Process', *Am. J. Sociol.,* 66, 1961, p.326.
50. See V. Navarro, 'Women in Health Care', *New Eng. J. Med.,* 229, 8, 1975, pp.398-402.
51. Source, *DHSS Health Personnel and Social Service Statistics, 1975.* Precise figures cannot be given because the recordings under-estimate the contribution of women. About 25 per cent of the overseas-born doctors are estimated to come from the 'Old Commonwealth and South Africa'.
52. See, for example, the Todd Report, op. cit.
53. For a recent account of the position of overseas doctors, see Community Relations Commission, *Doctors from Overseas: A Case for Consultation,* London, 1976. For a historical review of the position of women doctors, see Parry and Parry, op. cit., pp.162-86, and for the current position, M. A. Elston, 'Women in Medicine: Whose Problem?'—paper presented to the British Sociological Association's Annual Conference, Manchester, 1976.
54. In one Scottish area recently visited by the author, the number of registrar and houseman posts recognised for post-graduate training purposes was only half the number required to run the area's hospitals.
55. See, for example, R. Barron and G. M. Norris, 'Sexual Divisions and the Dual Labour Market', in D. Leonard-Barker and S. Allen (eds.), *Dependence and Exploitation in Work and Marriage,* Longmans, London, 1976, pp.47-69.
56. By 1963, house officers had enjoyed salary increases of infinity or 1,600 per cent under the NHS, depending upon whether they used to get nothing or

£50 per annum. Forsyth, op. cit., p.27.

57. Godber, op. cit., p.29.

58. Stevens, op. cit., p.143.

59. Source for these figures and for others unless otherwise stated in DHSS Statistics and Research Division.

60. The failure of the Ministry of Health to impose drastic reductions in the number of Registrars and Senior Registrars as an economy measure and to solve the post-war career bottleneck has been fully documented by Eckstein, op. cit., 1960, pp.112-25. Some restriction was brought in; the number of Senior Registrars in England and Wales fell between 1949 and 1959 from 1,430 to 931 and did not exceed the 1949 level till 1969. The number of Registrars rose in contrast between 1949 and 1959 from 1,523 to 2,787, and by 1969 was almost three times the 1949 figure at 4,467. Restrictions on the Registrar establishment were brought in in 1967 and the increase has slowed down. Thus, in 1967, there were 4,416 Registrars and in 1973, 4,834. During the same period, the number of senior house posts increased from 3,939 6,679. The latter have now become subject to stricter control and it may be anticipated that the non-training grades, i.e. clinical assistant and hospital practitioner grades will show a greater expansion in the future.

61. J. Parkhouse, 'Medical Manpower', *The Lancet,* 11 September 1976, pp.566-7.

62. See Ministry of Health, *Report of Joint Working Party on the Medical Staffing Structure in the Hospital* (Platt Report), HMSO, London, 1961 and DHSS *Report of Working Party on the Responsibilities of the Consultant Grade* (Godber Report), HMSO, London, 1969.

63. I am indebted to Chris Ham for providing evidence of these points from his study of the history of the Leeds Regional Hospital Board, currently being carried out.

64. Parkhouse, op. cit.

65. See B. Abel-Smith and K. Gales, *British Doctors at Home and Abroad,* Occasional Papers on Social Administration No. 8, 1964, for a study of emigration in the 1960s, and O. Gish, *Doctor Migration and World Health,* Occasional Papers on Social Administration, No. 43, 1971, for an international perspective.

66. *British Medical Journal,* 1 January 1976, p.3.

67. B. Senewiratne, 'The Emigration of Doctors: A Problem for the Developing and the Developed Countries', *The Lancet,* 15 and 22 March 1975, pp.618-20 and 669-71.

68. See Gunawardena and Lee, this volume.

69. For this reason the attempt of the new Central Manpower Committee to redistribute Senior Registrars, which are unequivocally *training* posts, unlike Registrarships, as a way of solving the *staffing* problems of peripheral hospitals is unpopular with junior doctors. Not only are such posts remote from influential patrons essential for future promotions but, while the greater responsibility carried resulting from lower staffing levels may be good learning experience, it leaves less time for study and research. The Godber Report, op. cit., paragraph 21, stressed that doctors in training should not be burdened with inappropriate clinical work and called for increases in consultant staffing.

70. There is insufficient space to trace the complex course of negotiations since 1970 leading up to the form of contract agreed in 1975. Briefly, between 1970 and 1974, negotiations centred around the principle of an 80-hour contract with extra duty allowances, and subsequently for a 40- (or 44-) hour basic contract. The more recent militancy, during 1976, has related to the implementation of this contract under the terms of the Labour government's

pay policy. These negotiations in particular were conducted by the junior doctors themselves (though they were not a united body).

71. Supplement to 5th Report of Review Body on Doctors and Dentists Remuneration, 19 September 1975.

72. The Junior Hospital Doctors' Association was founded as a 'ginger group' within the BMA in 1966, becoming an autonomous organisation in 1969. It currently has about 5,500 members out of approximately 17,500 junior doctors. The policies pursued by the 'junior doctors' since 1970 have been partly those of the JHDA through an uneasy alliance with the BMA juniors.

73. The Regional Hospital Consultants and Specialists' Association was founded in 1948 as a counter to the London-dominated BMA. (Ironically the same reasons for which the BMA was founded in 1832 as the Provincial Medical and Surgical Association as a counter to the Royal Colleges.) The prefix 'Regional' was dropped in January 1974. It was not a significant force until about 1970, when it gained recruits by pursuing a militant line specifically for consultants. Its membership rose by 250 per cent between 1972 and 1974, and it currently claims some 5,000 members, about 40 per cent of consultants. The support for the HCSA's more militant tactics in 1974 after the breakdown of the Owen Working Party forced the BMA to follow suit and condone working to rule in January 1975.

74. The BMA as a negotiating body involves the form of several largely autonomous craft committees; namely the General Medical Services Committee of General Practitioners, the Central Committee for Hospital Medical Services for Consultants, and latterly, the Central Committee for Community Medicine and the Hospital Junior Staffs Committee.

75. *British Medical Journal Supplement,* 2, 1972, p.45.

76. *British Medical Journal Supplement,* 27 April 1974, p.158.

77. H. Eckstein, *The English Health Service: Its Origins, Structures and Achievements,* Harvard University Press, Cambridge, Mass., 1958; M. Foot. *Aneurin Bevan, 1945-60,* Paladin, London, 1975, pp.106-215.

78. *A Review of the Medical Services in Great Britain,* Royal College of Physicians, London, 1962.

79. Ministry of Health, *The Administrative Structure of Medical and Related Services in England and Wales* (First Green Paper), HMSO, London, 1968.

80. Department of Health and Social Security, *The Future Structure of the National Health Service* (Second Green Paper), HMSO, London, 1970.

81. See *British Medical Journal,* 16 May 1970, p.375.

82. P. Draper, G. Greenholm and G. Best, 'The Organisation of Health Care: A Critical View of the 1974 Reorganisation of the National Health Service' in D. Tuckett (ed.), *An Introduction to Medical Sociology,* Tavistock, London, 1976, p.274.

83. This debate was sparked off by the GMC's request in 1970 for an annual retention fee in place of registration for life to solve its financial problems and led to the establishment of the Merrison Committee in 1972. *Report of the Committee of Inquiry into the Regulation of the Medical Profession,* HMSO, London, 1975.

84. R. G. S. Brown, S. Griffin and S. C. Heywood, *New Bottles: Old Wine?,* Institute of Health Studies, University of Hull, pp.50-2.

85. Ibid., pp.116-17.

86. Ibid., pp.101-2.

87. Department of Health and Social Security, *Management Arrangements for the Reorganised National Health Service*, HMSO, London, 1973.
88. *British Medical Journal*, 25 November 1972, p.444.
89. See Brown *et al.*, op. cit., pp.101-2 and p.116, and G. Cummings, 'The role of the clinician in the reorganised NHS—an eye witness account', *Hospital and Health Service Review*, 6, 72, June 1976, pp.192-5 and 7, 72, July 1976, pp.227-30. For a discussion of the problems facing the doctors elected to represent their often far-from-united colleagues, see Brown *et al.*, op. cit., and for an administrators' view, *A Review of the Management of the Reorganised NHS, 1976*, undertaken by a working party of chief administrators of health authorities. For a discussion of the role of the community physician, see Towell, this volume.
90; Cogwheel divisions are broad speciality-based groups, coming together in the Medical Executive Committee set up to co-ordinate hospital work. The name 'Cogwheel' refers to the cover design of the reports in question, e.g. Ministry of Health, *First Report of Joint Working Party on the Organisation of Medical Work in Hospitals*, HMSO, London, 1969. A report of their work prior to re-organisation can be found in Department of Health and Social Security, *Second Report of Joint Working Party on the Organisation of Medical Work in Hospitals*, HMSO, London, 1972; G. McLachlan (ed.), *In Low Gear? An examination of 'Cogwheels'*, Nuffield Provincial Hospitals Trust, London, 1971; and Brown *et al.*, op. cit., pp.47-51. There was a special report on the relationships between Cogwheel Divisions and the reorganised structure: Department of Health and Social Security, *Third Report of Joint Working Party on the Organisation of Medical Work in Hospitals*, HMSO, London, 1974.
91. S. Green, 'Professional/Bureaucratic Conflict: The Case of the Medical Profession in the National Health Service', *Sociological Review*, 1,23, February 1975, p.132. Also S. Green, *The Hospital: An Organisational Analysis*, Blackie, Glasgow, 1974.
92. See P. Draper and P. Smart, 'Social Science and Health Policy in the United Kingdom: some contributions of the social sciences to the bureaucratisation of the National Health Service', *Int. J. Health Services*, 4, 1974, pp.453-70.
93. As Johnson, this volume, has pointed out, patients have never been 'passive'. However, patient activity is often regarded as a problem by doctors, rather than as an essential part of care.
94. Department of Health and Social Security, *Democracy in the National Health Service, Membership of Health Authorities*, HMSO, London, 1974.
95. Parry and Parry, op. cit., p.212. See also Stevens, op. cit. This blaming of the NHS (or the DHSS) is seen very clearly in the 'Policy of Despair' BMJ leader discussed above.
96. Bevan, op. cit., pp.110-11.

Acknowledgement

This paper draws on material from the *Medical Careers Study* currently being carried out by Malcolm Johnson and the author, funded by the Social Science Research Council.

3 ACCESS AND EFFICIENCY IN MEDICAL CARE: A CONSIDERATION OF ACCIDENT AND EMERGENCY SERVICES

Arthur Gunawardena and Kenneth Lee

In any attempt to explore the difficulties and tensions in the NHS, accident and emergency (A and E) services provide, perhaps more than any other sector of the Service, something of a test case. In one respect they share with family practitioner services the distinction of being viewed as 'cornerstones', in as much as their removal would immediately undermine the structure of the present NHS. In a real sense, A and E services epitomise everything that is believed valuable in the NHS visibly demonstrating man's concern for his fellow being. By making an instant response to the unpredictability and uncertainty of illness or accident, these services provide support at a potentially critical moment in an individual's life. In this way, the 'cornerstone' becomes not simply a key feature of the NHS but more evidently a key support to the well-being of the community.

Yet in other respects, to make the dichotomy explicit, these very services have been viewed throughout their history as 'casualties' of the NHS, in as much as the observed reality fails to match the expectations and images projected of it. The 'Cinderella' label—the 'poor' relation of the NHS—has too often been attached to both A and E departments and ambulance services alike for the conflicts and tensions surrounding their objectives and current practices to be ignored. It is, therefore, to these apparent conflicts and the underlying tensions they create that this essay is addressed, in the belief that by so doing it will also offer lessons about society and our present approaches to social policy.

The manner of provision of accident and emergency services within the NHS has not been without its critics in recent times, as witnessed, for example, in the increasing number of official and independent enquiries conducted into its practice.[1] In part this increasing exposure to public debate may be attributed to its unique position within the NHS—as the 'shop-window' by which the public judges its hospital services—though other reasons are readily advanced for the current expression of concern and anxiety. The sources of these concerns are several. On one level it has been argued that improvements in the organisation and delivery of emergency health care have not kept pace with advances in medical technology and know-how, a school of thought emanating in large part from within a section of the medical profession itself.[2] Paradoxically, the medical profession has not been without its own internal conflicts as to the status it wishes to give to those of its members who work in this arena. At another level the disenchantment arises with consumers who argue that the gap between current levels of provision and their expectations is forever widening. In yet another, and more general, sense the root cause for this discontent is attributed to the NHS itself in its aim to be both comprehensive and free.

The debate, however, is not purely one of under-finance, in relation to what can and cannot be done. To see it as such is certainly to miss the point. Rather it is that accident and emergency services are increasingly seen not just as 'casualty centres' of the NHS but as important providers of primary care. Thus they become the victim of conflicts and tensions within the medical profession itself as to what the role should be, and who should perform it. In turn, this tension between 'critical care' medicine and 'primary care' medicine highlights a wider dilemma, for seemingly the A and E section of medicine appears to be giving more prominence to consumer opinion. The result is, perhaps only too predictably, seen in practice as an uncomfortable, and often unwilling, accommodation of conflicting roles and relationships, not least those between providers and consumers. This essay, then, presents a critique of these various conflicts, with a view both to clarifying the basic principles upon which the future development of these services might be based and to identifying what planning strategies might be appropriate. Two familiar considerations will be underlying the discussion: firstly, emergency services are embedded in a wider health care delivery system such that a recognition of the degree to which resources compete with or complement each other is a necessary prerequisite to planning their future direction; secondly, and at the broadest level, there are important policy trade-offs between prevention and treatment and that whilst attention has been in practice directed in favour of treatment the importance of prevention must be asserted in future policy formation.

Historical Perspective

Although accident and emergency services are often seen in many commentators' eyes as being synonymous with 'casualty departments', the reality can be more accurately viewed as a collection of services, both hospital- and community-based, largely independently organised and planned, offering a variety of skills and tasks, and with, until recently, few genuine attempts at improving their co-ordination. Yet, placed in a historical perspective there can be little doubt that those arms of the NHS established to respond to the 'unpredictable and uneven incidence of illness' have developed a separate viability out of all recognition to their humble beginnings. For instance, the ambulance service has seen in the last thirty years a movement from voluntary co-operation to a full-time employed service, accompanied by significant advances in the training of ambulancemen and in vehicle and equipment provision and, albeit more recently, in establishing national standards.[3] Criticisms where they have come have not been addressed at these developments as such, but rather at their pace of implementation, often referring by comparison to the increasing use of paramedical personnel in both Eastern Europe (the feldsher) and North America (the emergency medical technician).

This movement towards a professional identity has perhaps been even more marked in the hospital sector where, since the nineteenth century, forms of medical provision known as casualty work had developed in close association with out-patient clinics. Increasingly this emphasis had been viewed with some misgivings although until the late 1950s there were few cries over the state of affairs.[4] An enquiry carried out by the Nuffield Provincial Hospitals Trust and its publication in 1960 stands out as a landmark in the study of A and E services in terms of highlighting concern for the 'inadequate' pattern and scale of hospital-based services then existing. This report was closely followed by the Platt Committee Report (1962), its major contribution being to recommend changing the focus of interest from 'casualty' work to 'accident and emergency' work, through improved medical staffing of major accident and emergency units and through its desire to see larger but fewer A and E units set up with adequate staffing at all times. Though this thinking has been shown to have limitations in a number of significant respects,[5] its emphasis upon the creation of large units and the movement towards a speciality of emergency medicine stand out as important contributions. The trend towards concentrating hospital resources into designated A and E departments open for 24 hours each day and based on wide catchment areas has continued unabated, though it is probably correct to say that it was not so much prompted by likely economies of internal scale as by notions of medical viability and continuity of care. The second major change it prompted was the movement towards full-time consultants in A and E work though this innovation was to be delayed for another decade.

Set against an increasing groundswell of opinion in favour of the increasing professionalisation of A and E work, the problems facing the NHS today in this field may be regarded as less obvious. Yet it is precisely the pursuit of this goal, punctuated by advances made in response to individual pressures and crises, that has side-tracked the debate away from the crucial issues. Thus concern has regularly been expressed either at the level of consultant and other categories of staffing, or in terms of the 'casual attender', with little or no debate arising around the basic question—where does A and E care fit into any given overall system of medical care? In other words, the danger of a piecemeal approach is that it pre-empts discussion of the more fundamental issue: to identify the most appropriate and effective response to accident and emergency situations. Now, it could be speculated that there is nothing intrinsically characteristic of A and E care that distinguishes it from other branches of medical care or, indeed, successfully separates emergency patients from non-emergency cases. To pursue this line of reasoning would be to question the validity of the criteria frequently used to demarcate A and E from the remainder of the NHS, namely those conditions however caused which require immediate intensive therapy based on the criterion of medical diagnosis. The proponent and critic are equally forced back on to definitional issues and upon the imprecision with which the terms 'accident' and 'emergency' are frequently deployed.

Workable Definitions of Accidents and Emergencies

By way of introduction, one might volunteer the definition that 'accident cases' are those who suffer from recent injury, and 'emergencies' are those taken suddenly ill; and that in both cases these only relate to those patients who require hospital treatment and cannot be treated outside of the hospital setting. Under such terms, the hospital's A and E department and the Ambulance Service's emergency service could be regarded as possessing the skills of a 'speciality in time', as a 24-hour service open seven days a week. However, such a definition can readily be seen to be too restrictive in describing the work of either the hospital or ambulance-based emergency services. Thus, for example, the 'self-referral' is identified, defined as an attender who demands medical facilities at an A and E department without prior medical diagnosis. Some of these can be attendances of a life- or limb- threatening nature. The Platt Report commented that 'self-referrals are not necessarily trivial, for 61 per cent of them were asked to reattend A and E departments or outpatient departments and fewer than 25 per cent were discharged after the first visit'.[6] Though this is less of a feature in today's national statistics, a substantial proportion of self-referrals are still admitted or asked to re-attend the A and E department or out-patient clinic. Recent data obtained from a large A and E department in the North of England reveals that approximately one-third of all self-referrals were given follow-up hospital treatment either as in-patients or out-patients.[7]

Yet, contrary to the original idea behind the establishment of accident and emergency departments, namely to discourage the 'casual attender' and to foster a role for the department as a location solely for the treatment of urgent medical needs, it is evident that substantial numbers of people use the department for the treatment of non-urgent problems. The word 'urgent' of course has several connotations, but whichever connotation is attached, it is somewhat academic to the hospital doctor who is required to respond. For example, the Casualty Surgeons Association conceded that the term 'emergency' may have to be defined in terms of 'circumstances in which incapacity from injury or illness occurs and do not imply that the diagnosis is necessarily one requiring immediate intensive therapy'.[8] This trend of thought—contrary to the traditional line of argument—may have been forced upon this section of the medical profession if only because it is vir-tually impossible for a hospital to turn away a patient unexamined—particularly as the onus is commonly placed upon junior medical staff fulfilling a six-month training post, prior to climbing the ladder to a clinical speciality.

Despite, therefore, a disapproval in some quarters as to the 'triviality' of certain cases—loosely equated with the casual attender—the acceptance of non-acute care into the grand design of A and E hospital centres is perpetuated, and is indeed endorsed in some impor-tant quarters.[9] For instance, the Casualty Surgeons Association in commenting upon a sub-set of the self-referrals—designated as 'casual attenders'—remarked that '. . . whether such attenders are "wrong attenders" is less important than their reasons for not seeing, or being unable to see, a GP in the first place '.[10] But to view the phenomenon of self-referral in terms of the failings of GP services is to miss a vital sign. For the picture is replicated in other countries where the family practitioner is neither so prevalent nor so relevant. For example, it would appear that despite significant systemic differences in medical care provision, the picture currently presented in the United States accurately reflects our own—'The Hospital Emergency Department is confronted with a pot pourri of patient problems ranging from life-threatening emergencies to the "worried well".'[11]

The key to the whole issue lies in the motivation of consumers to seek 'help' from the A and E department. Given that all self-referral cases have made a lay diagnosis before presenting themselves to the hospital it is only to be expected that the utilisation of A and E services will provide the medical profession with a wider frame of reference than purely clinical criteria.[12] Hence, perceptions of illness, particularly its social causes and manifestations, may figure more prominently than professional notions of severity of illness. To indict consumers as 'casual users' or 'abusers' of NHS resources is both to expect consumers to make a medical rather than a social diagnosis and to argue that resources should be provider- rather than consumer-oriented. But it cannot be polarised that way. The A and E department is increasingly open to both client-initiated cases, self-referrals, and profession-initiated cases, GP referrals. When one section of the medical profession wishes to open the door to cases of minor trauma in order to avoid 'unnecessary suffering and delay in healing and unnecessary expense on drugs and dressings',[13] then the long-standing argument regarding the casual attender becomes largely redundant.

Once it is accepted, as increasingly appears to be the case, that all those who demand medical care from (hospital and ambulance) A and E services must be accommodated—in the sense that a response is required—the functions of the services broaden to include almost all forms of medical care. Though it may be uncomfortable to accept this reality, understandably in view of its implications for the rationality of resource use and for the distribution of health care, at least it will have been a response to consumer preferences, as revealed by their demand patterns. As Baderman, a prominent spokesman of the field said:

> To make a definition at the beginning too narrow as to severity or extent of acute clinical conditions, or too narrow in defining it for only organic clinical conditions, is not only to ignore recent trends— and a very significant non-organic proportion of the A and E case load, as it does in fact present itself in our present society—but also to preclude a more imaginative approach to organising present A and E, and planning for the future.[14]

In a climate where the whole medical tradition is geared towards compartmentalising medical care it is not perhaps surprising to observe that the case-mix and severity/acuteness criterion has been applied to defining A and E services. But in reality this criterion can only be applied strictly when medical care is sought beyond primary care, and in circumstances where the general practitioner is the consumer's sole entry point into the

NHS. Once the hospital's A and E department becomes progressively opened-up as a primary mode of access to medical care, and hence alternative to GP referral, the perceptions of a single medical group can no longer determine the utilisation patterns of particular services. The picture then becomes one of how best to handle the diversity and severity of cases presented and it is here that the importance of *triage* emerges. The concept of *triage*—originally a French word meaning 'sorting' and borrowed directly from the armed forces—is relevant to both A and E departments and ambulance services in selecting and treating patients. Although the military connotation of triage was in selecting patients according to military priority, the concept has in recent years come to be used in a different way in some A and E departments: the selection and treatment of the more serious patient.[15] What visible evidence is there then of changes in the utilisation rates of particular emergency services?

Table 1:   Out-patients: Accident and Emergency Departments and Total Numbers (England, per thousand population)

	Attendance of New Cases (Accident and Emergency Department)	Total A and E Attendances	Out-patients Department Attendances (New Cases)
1956	114.6	270.0	163.1
1961	137.6	291.0	165.6
1966	149.4	295.0	158.9
1971	170.8	284.9	168.1
1975	180.1	273.9	150.6

Sources: Various Annual Reports of the Ministry of Health and the Department of Health and Social Security, 1956-75.

Before documenting some of the salient features in the changing volume and distribution of patient demands' upon A and E services, it is relevant to note the pathways patients take in their attempts to gain access to the medical care system. In so doing, the distinction can be made between the growth of accident and emergency cases *per se* (defined in some technical sense) and the relative growth of demand for A and E as a form of general medical care. The first aspect of growth will likely be rooted in the underlying aetiology of illness and hence revealed by demographic and epidemiological data; whereas explanation for the second aspect of growth may be more likely found through organisational data and the determinants discovered by analysing the process by which consumers substitute hospital services for GP services or indeed self-medication. Table 1 gives an indication as to how the total growth of demand for hospital A and E services has increased over a twenty-year period. However, these figures only show that there is a general increasing trend of new cases over the period and are less helpful in isolating the contributing factors to this trend. Yet there is some patchy evidence to the effect that the case-mix and the composition of the type of incident has been changing over the period.[16] It has also been noticed that there is a variation in case-mix geographically.[17] For example, Caro suggests that, especially in large busy departments in certain metropolitan areas, the emphasis often falls more on medical and surgical emergencies and trauma may only take third place.[18] The significance of this changing composition of case-mix is that it supports the hypothesis that at least some part of the growth in demand can be attributed both to organisational features of the delivery system and to the exercise of consumer preferences. In this respect, Table 1 raises interesting questions for it shows that the growth rate in new attendances at the A and E department is not reflected in the growth rate of total A and E attendances, but rather the reverse. Thus, the decreasing number of total patients seen in the departments shows that increasing numbers of cases have been discharged on the first visit, which, in turn, is at least suggestive that an increasing proportion of patients are less urgent or more 'trivial' cases. That increased utilisation of A and E departments is not also revealed in total new out-patient attendances is also at least suggestive that the growth is less to be explained in terms of changes in morbidity as in changes of either an organisational nature or of consumer wishes.

The implication of this growth in demand is twofold. First, it strongly suggests that the modes of service provision commonly assumed desirable and offered by providers have become increasingly contested by consumers. Paradoxically, the exercise of consumer 'rights' will have given way to shifts in the distribution of health care, in as much as those patients using hospital A and E facilities as a substitute for GP services may possess more facilities for access than others and thereby effectively gain a wider choice in health care. On one reading, therefore, the growth factor in the A and E services is a manifestation of more important underlying issues in the wide field of general medical or primary care. Second, the picture can be viewed as a dilemma between a 'critical care model' of emergency care which argues for the concentration of resources and the development of hospital

centres of excellence; and a 'primary care model' which, by incorporating minor non-traumatic ailments, argues for 'despecialisation' and
routine medical services; it is to a consideration of each of these models
that the essay now turns.

The Place of Accident and Emergency Services in the Primary Care Model

If it is difficult in theoretical terms to make a clear distinction between
the role of general practitioner services and of hospital services in accident and emergency care, in practice the distinction appears even more
blurred when consumers view them both as primary access points to
medical care. Indeed, historically, hospital casualty departments in
urban and inner-city areas have long been providers for all forms of care.
On a purely technical point a demarcation is frequently made in surgical cases as between 'major' trauma, where hospital-based medical
investigations and treatments are required and 'minor' trauma, where
such facilities are not required. One might imagine that this criterion
could also be applied to medical cases yet, under operational circumstances, patient flow patterns do not readily conform to the meeting of
professional definitions.

Although the exercise of consumer choice for hospital A and E
department, or GP surgery, or health centre services is as yet ill-defined,
a number of factors can be readily postulated. In the first place, consumer preference patterns are determined both by their knowledge of
the availability of GP services and by their perceptions of the quality of
care that might be available to treat their illness or injury.[19] This percep-
tion is, in turn, conditioned by their own experiences, hearsay and the
influence of the lay-referral system (family, friends, workmates) as
much as by the organisational features (appointments systems,
deputising services). Secondly, it can be hypothesised that consumers'
preferences are influenced by the resource implications they face in
terms of travel and time costs which, in turn, are a function of the
relative proximity, mode of travel and congestion features of the hospital department compared with the GP's surgery. This second set of
considerations helps to explain the 'peakiness' of A and E department
activity by time of day and week, as shown in the incidence of 'com-
muter demand' from people who work a long way from their GP, and
by week of year reflecting the seasonal pattern of holidays. Finally,
account must be taken of the influence of a third party such as a police-
man or an ambulanceman who takes a decision on behalf of the patient
and whose preference may well be for the facilities of the nearest
hospital, or the nearest designated A and E hospital.

This link between primary services (particularly general practitioner services) and accident and emergency services can either be expressed in terms of their *substitutability* or in terms of their *complementarity*. The health professionals' traditional model of the NHS would emphasise the complementarity aspects, whereas today in many settings substitutability exists because of the exercise of choice of care by patients. In such circumstances the institutional frameworks are inevitably strained, for GP services not only then compete with A and E services but also compete for customers.[20]

The *complementarity* aspect may be considered as follows. It has been repeatedly acknowledged that GPs cannot provide comprehensive medical treatment which embraces everything from minor non-traumatic illness to major traumatic situations. In some instances, GPs use the A and E department as a means of seeking a second opinion and, in others, to refer those patients who may require various kinds of radiological or pathological investigations which are increasing in sophistication and cost, and which may also need further care through in-patient treatment. In such cases GP and A and E services function complementarily once the GP has taken the initial decision. However, in order for this to be so, contact must first be made between the patient and the GP, which under many circumstances may prove difficult. Many kinds of human or physical barriers can exist between the patient and GP which may lead towards self-referral, 999 ambulance calls, or police referral direct to the A and E department. Thus it seems that a crucial factor in the successful coexistence of GP—A and E services is identifying who is to do the initial 'sorting out' of cases, and when and where this is to occur. Given that at present this act of 'sorting out' is carried out by a variety of groups in a variety of settings, the question of substitution becomes self-evident.

The notion of *substitutability* as between primary care and emergency care, i.e. that the role of one can be appropriately performed by the services of another, has been generated in large part by two factors: (a) patients' preferences in the choice of care; and (b) the conscious channelling of cases to A and E departments as a result of the pressures upon GP services; leading to the so-called misuse and 'abuse' of hospital facilities. As witnessed earlier, increased utilisation of A and E departments has prompted much criticism of late and has given rise to various publicity campaigns aimed at correcting what has come to be regarded as an unwelcome trend. Similar campaigns have been launched to 'educate' the public in the use of their GP in the belief that 'a major problem is to detrivialise the demand on the service, especially but not

exclusively in general practice'.[21] The irony of such campaigns is that
their argument contrasts sharply with increasing documentation on consumer reluctance to seek medical treatment for specific conditions,
such as the threat of a heart attack, where pressure is in the reverse direction to educate the general public to seek earlier medical attention in
order to improve the outcomes of medical intervention after the onset
of the attack. The dilemma for the medical profession is to induce some
patients to refrain from presenting their 'trivial' cases whilst simultaneously encouraging other clients to give the doctors the earliest possible
indication of their pathology. Though this would appear on one reading
to be a simple case of selecting the right deterrents and incentives, on
another reading it rests on the questionable supposition that the patient
is in a position to draw a clear medical distinction between 'trivia' and
'severity'. Furthermore, one might argue that even if the patient was in
a position to comply with such a neat organisational solution, this may
well run counter to his wishes.

The rationale for this 'contradictory' behaviour by the consumer can
be sought by attempting to examine possible reasons for such behaviour.
On a theoretical basis one could argue that the consumer consciously
searches for alternatives/substitutes in order to broaden the choices
available to him. Accessibility to medical treatment and personal perceptions regarding the quality of care are two major factors for him. At
the same time commentators are also increasingly asking whether the
present changes in GP organisation are having a noticeable influence
upon consumer behaviour. Currently GP services are marked by three
particular features: the growing reliance on deputising services; the
emergence of appointments systems; and the growth of group practice.
In these changing circumstances of both patient demand and physician
supply, the traditional role of the GP in the field of primary care stands
only to be challenged. Although the Gillie Report on General Practice
in 1963 [22] maintained that the family doctor's personal knowledge of
his patients equips him as 'the essential intermediary in the trans-
mission of specialist skills to the individual', its indispensability is now
continuously contested as illustrated by the noted increasing trend of
self-referral. Conway,[23] in studying the attendance of emergency medical patients at a district general hospital in five separate periods between
1973 and 1975, showed that over half the patients had referred themselves, and that of those subsequently admitted 37 per cent were
self-referred. Patel[24] had found even higher self-referral rates in survey-
ing a teaching hospital's activity between 1968 and 1970 and revealed
that about 15 per cent of those interviewed who had visited the

department had done so as a result of the GP appointments system. Furthermore, another 10 per cent had said that they had attended hospital due to the non-availability of their GPs, whilst 30 per cent of patients were of the view that GP services were not generally or readily available at other than surgery hours. In contrast, another recent study[25] found that the alleged case of a high positive association between A and E use and the presence of appointments systems and/or use of deputising services was not statistically proven. Thus the picture is still not clear and the research evidence is suggestive rather than conclusive. But it is not unreasonable to infer that in the minds of some members of the public the introduction of appointments systems necessarily creates delay in seeing the doctor and may even reduce the time the doctor devotes to each patient.

In contrast, the use of deputising services by GPs would seem to change the quality of the service given, though in what direction is as yet uncertain. But it does appear that these two factors (appointments systems, deputising services) have had an overall effect, and that is to drive a wedge between GP and patient. Whether this is a permanent and ever-widening gap between the GP and the patient, affecting the nature and quality of their relationship, is an issue that can only be debated against the background of changing consumer attitudes on the one hand and the sophistication of medical technology on the other. What it does reveal is that the GP concept in its traditional form may be in need of revision and clarification if general practice is to sustain its role as the premier access point to emergency medicine and, indeed, to primary care itself.

The Place of Accident and Emergency Services in the Critical Care Model

Discussion in the previous section on the increasing primary care character of much of today's hospital A and E department work load must not mask the department's function in critical care medicine. The functional links between the A and E department, hospital clinical firms such as neurology, cardiology, thoracic surgery, and diagnostic services of pathology and radiology illustrate very clearly that life- and limb-threatening conditions call for certain types of specialist technology (medical as well as non-medical) constituting a separate and distinctive form of care. Indeed the main spur in creating A and E departments since the Platt Report has been the need of a specialised form of emergency medical services (EMS) to care for the critically injured, its most dramatic form being the provision of care in the event of major disasters. And although major disasters are expected to be infrequent phenomena, the critical care function remains the essential justification for A and E departments.

The need for an efficient EMS is justified on a number of grounds. Aldridge[26] claims that the EMS deal for most part with the most socially valuable section of the community and certainly the most economically valuable, whilst the Platt Report in 1962 noted that one-eighth of the community's total working life is lost among males as measured by death before the age of 65 (and no estimates are available on loss of work-time due to non-fatal injuries). Apart from the educational activities of health services on prevention, i.e. to minimise the risk of accidental injury or disease, the existence of EMS is seen as a form of insurance to minimise the consequences of this loss. But unfortunately, unlike other forms of insurance the resources diverted to perform this insurance function against the risks of accidental injury or death are so specific that from the point of view of society they are perceived to lie idle or remain under-utilised, and hence *high-cost* providers, a characteristic seemingly shared by other (exclusively) emergency cover, e.g. fire services. It is within this context that the possibility is opened up of these same EMS resources becoming available at certain times of the day or week for the provision of services to patients who are not critically ill. Suddenly it appears that self-referral cases, the 'casual attenders', the 'non-urgent' cases, become an important asset to the A and E service, in delivering *low-cost* medicine at high levels of utilisation. Thus on this reading the self-referral process and primary care aspects of the department's work should not simply be accepted but positively encouraged.

However, on a wider reading, while it may be recognised in general terms that EMS do have a vital role to play in modern society the existing structure of the A and E service can only be reasonably evaluated against the fulfilment of defined objectives and functions. On one dimension A and E units are only a component in an emergency system where it is functionally related to other emergency services such as ambulance, fire and police services. On another dimension A and E is a part of EMS where the rest of the components include transportation of patients, medical investigation departments, in-patient services, clinics and rehabilitation services. And in this configuration GP services again become an integral part of the system.

One striking illustration of the way system linkages deserve closer attention in the UK is in terms of the alleged lack of 'on site' care. This has been known as a 'gap in medical care' or as a 'therapeutic vacuum',[27] and on-site treatment has been given strong support by the Medical

Practitioners' Union.[28] However, the argument continues as to whether it is a gap and, if so, as to who should fill the gap: should it be one of the traditional roles, e.g. a doctor or a nurse or an ambulanceman, or should it be a completely different newly conceptualised role—such as an Emergency Medical Technician (EMT)?[29] Indeed these questions can be asked in another perspective, i.e. whether the present piecemeal approach to A and E, in effect building up services in isolation from one another, is the right one? Undoubtedly the need for efficient EMS, especially where resources are coming under increasing pressure, calls for new approaches to the overall planning and organisation of this branch of medical care, and leads into the central debate surrounding medical manpower itself.

Resource Considerations and the Medical Manpower Issue

Apart from the debate surrounding the 'casual attender', there has been one other outstanding issue running through the whole history of A and E services—the staffing problem of A and E departments. As noted earlier, the Platt Report 'solution' was the creation of large-scale A and E departments, normally to serve populations of over 150,000 thereby encouraging the closure of small units in favour of concentrating A and E services within larger hospitals. Solutions to any problem of shortage in the A and E field have been largely conceived in terms of medical personnel, and thus the Platt policy was implemented, resulting in the reduction in the number of 'casualty units' in England and Wales from approximately 2,600 at the time of the Platt Report to about 680 by 1973.[30]

Yet, in this increasing movement towards larger but fewer A and E units two important manpower issues emerged: was A and E a speciality? and if so, who was qualified to undertake this task? Historically, A and E departments had been under the supervision of orthopaedic surgeons in the belief that the case-mix largely reflected the orthopaedic specialty. The Platt Report, for its part, had responded to the notion of doctor shortage by recommending that major A and E units employ up to three consultants on a part-time basis with further employment of other intermediate and junior staff based on local requirements. By so doing, it was expected that supervision could be provided for the junior staff by senior medical staff and that this would ease the problem of staffing.

Meanwhile, the momentum for a full-time consultant in the A and E department was gaining ground, if only because already there were misgivings about the low status that would be given to the department if those in charge were only to work part-time within it. In short, the dangers of the 'absentee landlord' were quickly apparent and casualty surgeons struggled for recognition of a new branch of medicine—a speciality in its own right—which would free itself from an image of orthopaedics' 'poor relation' which many thought had held it back for so long. As a result, although the part-time situation still exists in many parts of the country, there is an increasing trend towards the appointment of full-time consultants. To date, some one hundred appointments have already been made and a senior registrar training programme in accident and emergency medicine has also been approved.

At present, therefore, A and E now appears as a speciality since there are consultants in administrative charge and holding clinical responsibility on a full-time basis, with the official view tending to encourage the appointment of surgeons to A and E consultant posts. However, there is an accumulation of evidence that the content of A and E may be equally medically, as opposed to surgically, oriented. Such evidence offers support for a change in policy: more serious consideration should be given to appointing physicians[31] for A and E consultant posts or, even more radically, consultants with an interest in the primary care of a wide spectrum of cases. Certainly, the substantial body of survey data on A and E departments now available does support the view that the A and E work-load covers a very wide field and, thus, that A and E specialists must be seen to be either capable of handling every type of A and E case or at least qualified to co-ordinate work of a diversified nature. Is it not appropriate to ask, therefore, whether the historical dichotomy of physician and surgeon, on which the whole structure of hospital care is based, can provide a suitable framework for the development of A and E specialists?

The paradox is only too self-evident; if accident and emergency work requires the skill of the generalist in medicine rather than the specialist, then the concept of a speciality in 'emergency medicine' becomes vulnerable, and once again open to the 'low-prestige' problems of staff recruitment.[32] With the creation of A and E consultant posts a career structure has been established for junior staff and, as a result, one of the grave problems which the A and E service has faced hitherto might well disappear. But this remains to be seen, and is dependent in large part on changes yet to be seen in the medico-political circles of the NHS.

However, to view the issues and their resolution solely in terms of medical manpower is to overlook wider considerations. One practical issue which neatly illustrates the paradox identified above concerns the question as to who does (or should) perform the task of initially 'sorting' patients as they arrive at the hospital department. At present only doctors are authorised to perform this task;[33] the implication, indeed stipulation, that nurses cannot perform this function has been stressed in some quarters as one of the biggest obstacles to reorganising A and E departments.[34] Whether a clarification, or indeed a redefinition, of the medico-legal position is required is less at issue than that the nature of the work can be carried out effectively with different configurations of Health Service staff: the concepts of an emergency technician and a nurse practitioner with diagnostic responsibilities serve to illustrate that the debate about substitutability of skills between different health service staff groups—consultants, junior doctors, general practitioners, nurses, ambulancemen, to name no others—has scarcely begun.

A Rational Solution in Sight?

By focusing upon the problems of the 'casual attender' and 'medical staffing' this essay has attempted to show that observers so far have misguidedly overlooked the real problems underlying the current state of A and E services and, as a result, the prospects for their resolution.

On the demand side, it is of course within the province of the medical practitioner to appraise the urgency of a patient's medical needs. Admittedly many A and E cases are not urgent in their professional judgement, but this does not alter the fact that they are perceived as important by the patient. To assert, as some do, that the 'conditions' are not important to patients and to criticise patients for 'abusing' hospital services is misplaced. In part, it has been argued that the present pattern of self-referral may be more adequately explained as a changing historical process in the underlying aetiology of illness and in the changing determinants of demand for A and E services. The general belief implicit in many official documents that the presence of non-emergencies in A and E departments was a temporary phenomenon, and with suitably devised publicity campaigns would evaporate, has proved to be a fallacy.

A second fallacy has been in viewing problems largely in terms of a single supply factor, namely medical staffing. Unfortunately this specific manpower issue not only offered a lop-sided diagnosis of the broad issues associated with A and E services, but also side-tracked the development of ideas by failing to recognise fully changing consumer attitudes and perceived needs. In part, this may be explained by the reality that, amidst cries for greater rationality in resource usage, ambulance, hospital and family practitioner services remain at present in different domains at important levels of organisation. If the reorganisation of the NHS is to have any meaning in terms of developing a corporate and comprehensive approach to particular health care issues then, as argued elsewhere,[35] all components of emergency health care delivery require to be considered within a general system where their interrelationships are spelled out specifically. This would be a significant departure from simply viewing them as a collection of resources such as general practitioners, ambulancemen, casualty surgeons, health centres, communications, diagnostic facilities or hospital wards.

Indeed with more research effort we may yet find it is a fallacy to assume that in urban areas the use of A and E services by self-referrals is 'high-cost' medicine, or that in rural areas A and E services are 'uneconomic' to provide in community hospitals. The ready solution or blueprint applicable to all areas irrespective of demographical patterns, epidemiological profiles or consumer expectations may then turn out to be the pursuit of an illusion. More likely, planners may wish to consider a continuum of alternative strategies ranging from the re-education of the lay mind to accept the function of A and E departments for 'real' emergencies, to an acceptance by policy-makers of present utilisation patterns and the devising of policies accordingly.

Put bluntly, the demand for accident and emergency services has not turned out to be what those running the system would have chosen to make it, or indeed what they believe it should be. But this is inevitable since hospital A and E departments occupy the interface between the community and the provision of specialist treatment; though uncomfortable to some, this inevitably leads to the conclusion that the future planning of A and E services needs to be considered not only within the framework of both general primary care and critical care medicine, but also within the framework of patients' wishes and expectations.

If this suggests that A and E signifies Anything and Everything then so be it, for it cannot be otherwise. As a test case, the specifics of A and E services have illustrated clearly some of the fundamental dilemmas and conflicts implicit in the NHS and, moreover, in any system wishing to offer open access to comprehensive care. Against a back-cloth of limited resources, consumer behaviour and professional aspirations are pulling in different directions. This central fact emerges with crystal clarity in A and E services but, as other essays in this volume bear witness, it applies no less forcibly to other sections of the medical care system. As the terms of reference of the NHS Royal Commission make clear, the task ahead is an issue of *judgement* as to what should be the trade-offs between consumers, professionals and resources. What is thereby certain, and will remain so, is that there will be no easy solution either to A and E or to anything else. Equally certain is that medical care will have to live with Anything and Everything —in our time at least.

Notes

1. Nuffield Provincial Hospitals Trust, *Casualty Services and Their Settings,* Oxford University Press, 1960; Ministry of Health, *Accident and Emergency Services,* Report of the Sub-Committee, HMSO, 1962, Chairman Sir Henry Platt; British Medical Association, *Accident Services of Great Britain and Ireland,* Second Report of Review Committee, BMA House, Tavistock Square, London, 1965; British Orthopaedic Association, *Casualty Departments—The Accident Commitment,* Report by the British Orthopaedic Association, Accident and Emergency Services Sub-Committee, 1973; Department of Health and Social Security, *Accident and Emergency Services,* Government Observations on the Fourth Report of the Employment and Social Services Sub-Committee of the Expenditure Committee, Cmnd. 5886, HMSO, 1975.
2. As one prominent medical spokesman observed 'Scientific knowledge and methods of treatment of the injured have advanced enormously in the last fifty years. Where this advance has not been accompanied by improved organisation there has been no parallel improvement in the standard of care.' J. C. Scott, 'The Development of Accident Services', Accident and Emergency Services, *British Health Care and Technology,* Health and Social Services Journal/Hospital International, 1973, p.9.
3. See Department of Health and Social Security, *Organisation of Ambulance Services, Standard Measures of Service and Incentive Schemes,* HSC(IS)67, August 1974.
4. Some early discussions on the demand patterns for the services and the forms of the services to be provided can be found in T. G. Lowden, (i) 'The Casualty Department—The Work and the Staff', *The Lancet,* 16 June 1956, pp.955-6; (ii) 'The Casualty Department—Shortcomings and Difficulties', *The Lancet* 23 June 1956, p.1006; D. L. Crombie, 'A Casualty Survey', *Journal of the College of General Practitioners,* Vol. 2, 1959, pp.346-56.
5. See, for instance, D. B. Caro, 'The Casualty Surgeons Association', Proceedings of a Conference held at the Robert Jones and Agnes Hunt Orthopaedic Hospital, Oswestry, *Postgraduate Medical Journal,* Vol. 48, 1972, pp.260-1.
6. Ministry of Health (1962), op. cit., p.14.
7. The unpublished data arise from the preliminary results of a two-year Leeds-based study into accident and emergency services, conducted by the joint authors in conjunction with Mr D. H. Wilson, Consultant in charge of A and E services at the Leeds General Infirmary.
8. The Casualty Surgeons Association, *An Integrated Emergency Service,* Casualty Surgeons Association, 1973, p.4.
9. Not least in official circles, see HM(68)83, p.3, 'The obligation to "sort" casual attenders who present themselves direct to a hospital into those in need of hospital care and others not in need of hospital attention can be accepted by major accident and emergency departments, but is causing increasing difficulties at other hospitals.'
10. The Casualty Surgeons Association, 1973, op. cit., p.4.
11. R. E. Burnley and A. M. Sadler, 'Resources Utilised for the Care of Surgical Patients in the Emergency Department', *Medical Care,* December 1975, pp.1021-32.
12. This is most dramatically relevant in terms of the homeless. As Leighton

notes: 'a man living in a hostel or lodging house or on the street, tends to leave an illness or injury untreated for long periods of time before seeking medical attention and the usual pattern of care of the family doctor providing initial treatment with a referral to a hospital consultant if necessary and the use of a casualty in the event of accident, is often not appropriate for this group,' p.266; J. Leighton, 'Primary medical care for the homeless and rootless in Liverpool', *Hospital and Health Services Review,* August 1976, pp.266-7.

13. The Casualty Surgeons Association, 1973, op. cit., p.7.

14. Howard Baderman, *Accident and Emergency Services,* Kings Fund Centre Reprint No. 945, 1975.

15. For instance, ambulance services now classify patients into two categories of service—emergency and non-emergency—with urgent cases being a special sub-group of emergency work.

16. The Fourth Report from the House of Commons Expenditure Committee (1974) provides some information to support changing trends. For example, Road Traffic Accidents treated in hospitals (as in-patients) decreased during the period 1964-71. During the same period the rate of in-patient spells of cases of poisoning nearly doubled. For more information see Table 5, p.11.

17. Evidence available from published and unpublished surveys conducted in such different parts of the country as Glasgow, Leeds and London confirms this variation. See, for instance, R.·Pease, 'A Study of Patients in a London Accident and Emergency Deaprtment', *The Practitioner,* Vol. 211, November 1973, pp.634-8; and Leeds General Infirmary, 'Accident and Emergency Department—Statistical Memoranda 1976' (mimeographed), Leeds General Infirmary and Nuffield Centre for Health Services Studies, Leeds, 1976.

18. Caro, 1972, op. cit., p.261.

19. It has been suggested that patients are becoming more hospital-orientated due to visible signs of high-technology medical care available in hospital A and E departments. See T. Cull, 'The General Practitioners' View', *Postgraduate Medical Journal,* Vol. 48, 1972, p.266.

20. Cull, 1972, op. cit., p. 266.

21. See E. Wilkes, 'Unlimited demand—limited resources', *The Hospital and Health Services Review,* August 1976, p.275.

22. Ministry of Health, *The Field of Work of the Family Doctor,* Report of the Sub-Committee, HMSO, 1963, Chairman Mr A. Gillie, p.9.

23. H. Conway, 'Emergency Medical Care', *British Medical Journal,* 28 August 1976, pp.511-13.

24. A. R. Patel, 'Modes of Admission to Hospital: A Survey of Emergency Admissions to General Medical Unit', *British Medical Journal,* 30 January 1971, pp.281-3.

25. This study by Russell and Holohan (1974) attempts to quantify the contribution of a number of variables, including the presence of deputising services and appointment systems, towards the choice of care, i.e. GP services versus hospital A and E departments, in the field of minor trauma. Apart from the severe definitional problems in minor trauma, this area of illness is not the only one which has been the main subject of controversy over the casual attender. Arguably, it is the minor non-traumatic conditions which are as relevant to a study of this nature. See Appendix 36, Evidence to the Fourth Report from the Expenditure Committee. I. T. Russell, A. M. Holohan and J. H. Walker, Memorandum by the Medical Care Research Unit, University of Newcastle upon Tyne, 23 September 1973.

26. L. W. Aldridge, 'The Organisation and Staffing of Casualty Departments', Proceedings of a Conference held at the Robert Jones and Agnes Hunt

Orthopaedic Hospital, Oswestry, op. cit., pp. 251-94.

27. Report of an Inquiry by Special Panel, 'Gaps in Medical Care', *British Medical Journal Supplement,* 8 May 1971, pp.88-91. Appointed by the BMA Board of Science and Education.

28. Contained in a written memorandum submitted by the Medical Practitioners' Union to the House of Commons Expenditure Committee, 1974: House of Commons, Title—*Accident and Emergency Services,* Vols. I and II—'Fourth Report from the Expenditure Committee', HMSO, 1974, p.103.

29. The role of EMT and their relationship with the emergency medical service in the United States is described in Leslie R. Smith, 'From Ambulance Driver to EMT', *Hospitals,* Vol. 47, 16 May 1973, pp. 105-8. For a critical evaluation of the EMT system see Steve McDermott, 'Analysing the need for paramedics', *The Journal of Emergency Care and Transportation,* Vol. 5, No. 2, March/April 1976, pp.50-7.

30. These figures are quoted from Ministry of Health, 1962, op. cit., and House of Commons Expenditure Committee, op. cit., 1974.

31. HMSO, Cmnd. 5886, 1975, 'A positive effort should be made to recruit physicians as accident and emergency consultants where the case load renders such appointments particularly desirable', p.2.

32. This argument is predominant in Ministry of Health, op. cit., 1962; Proceedings of a Conference held at Robert Jones and Agnes Hunt Orthopaedic Hospital, Oswestry, op. cit., 1972, pp.249-94; and House of Commons Expenditure Committee, op. cit., 1974.

33. 'The responsibility for "sorting" patients who present themselves at a hospital into those who need hospital care and those who do not, cannot properly be carried out by other than a registered medical practitioner. It should not be placed on the nursing service.' See HM(68)83, 1968, p. 4.

34. Proceedings of a Conference held at the Robert Jones and Agnes Hunt Orthopaedic Hospital, Oswestry, 1972, op. cit., p.279.

35. For some exploration of the difficulties involved see U. Christiansen, 'Demand for Emergency Health Care and Regional Systems for Provision of Supply' in M. Perlman (ed.), *The Economics of Health and Medical Care,* 1974; and K. Lee, 'Management Sciences and the Organisation of Emergency Medical Services', First World Congress on Intensive Care, London, June 1974 (mimeographed).

4 PATIENTS: RECEIVERS OR PARTICIPANTS?

Malcolm L. Johnson

Unlike the retail trade, where an old dictum declares 'The customer is always right', in the professions he is only right when his professional adviser tells him so. The supremacy of knowldege and the monopoly of information which accompanies it has led the professions to the top of the social status and reward structure. It has also allowed them until recently to take an unquestioned dominant role in relation to their clients, who accept that the quality and integrity of their work is ensured by training, ethical standards and the corporate conscience of their professional associations. Despite the slings and arrows of a few assailants, even those as long ago and as witty and perceptive as Bernard Shaw on professions in his preface to *The Doctor's Dilemma*, little effective criticism has emerged. Until recently the professional—client relationship has remained in all its essential features in its traditional form.

Students of the professions have never been in doubt about the inclusion of medicine in this category. Indeed they have tended to put its practitioners in a special position as archetypes, embodying all the essential attributes. Thus the conventional interpretation of the doctor's professional and social position is one of wide autonomy and control over circumstances. The literature is a testament to this view. It goes back to Carr-Saunders[1] on this side of the Atlantic and Everett Hughes[2] on the other. The flow of studies since the war, whilst becoming increasingly radical in their commentary,[3] has maintained the division between an altruistically motivated provider of services and an ill-informed but grateful receiver. If anything, the more polemical writings have tended to further spell it out and reinforce the popular view.

Reassessment of the doctor—patient relationship has none the less begun. A number of changes within health care itself supply indicators of what is to come, whilst social scientists have now assembled a body of research and interpretation which casts new light on both the traditional and the new situation. The traditional view of the patient is one which cast him (or her) in the role of a receiver of expert services of a sort which he is incapable of evaluating and must therefore take on trust. Characteristically the patient is a supplicant whose main active involvement in diagnosis and prognosis is to provide information which is requested by the doctor. Judgements about his welfare and statements about his health are made by the doctor with some background knowledge of the individual, but with little or no discussion about their acceptability or appropriateness.

This construction of the consultation process in general practice is not a statement of the invariable manner of its conduct, but a broad generalisation against which recent thinking and movements can be set. In doing this, attention will be given to two seemingly related developments. The first is to be found in sociological studies of illness behaviour which during the past decade have given increasing attention to providing detailed accounts of actual behaviour at all stages of illness episodes. A shift in approach amongst some medical sociologists has provided a different level of analysis and fresh insight into how people think about illness and how they act out their perceptions of the situation before, during and after seeking medical help, if indeed they do so at all. Even the seemingly deferential role adopted by many in consulting their doctor can be seen as a calculated form of behaviour rather than mere passivity.

The object of this review of the sociological literature will be to show that the doctor—patient relationship is much more of a bargaining and interactive process than is commonly thought. This will lead on to discussion of the significance of the trend towards consumerism and greater knowledge and assertiveness amongst the consumer of goods and services. Part of that movement is the increasing sophistication of ordinary people in medical—as in other professional—matters. Amongst the manifestations of these changes is the strengthening of patient pressure groups and the emergence of community health councils as a real force in the health care field.

Thus, if there exists a long-established pattern of bargaining between patient and doctor which has frequently influenced or controlled medical management of illness, then in a climate of demand for greater consumer involvement, our traditional medical models clearly need re-examination. Health professionals will need to recognise these changes and respond to them in creative ways, if they are to maintain medicine as an effective service and retain the standing they have so long held in society.

Sociological Change

Sociological thinking which was dominated until the early sixties by the school of 'structural-functionalist' or systems theories and in Britain by empiricism, has expanded into a heterodox situation where several 'brands' of sociology uneasily coexist. The structural-functionalist view of the status of the professional is a clear reflection of the predominant accepted view of its time. Parsons[4] and Merton,[5] in their writings on the medical profession and on socially appropriate behaviour of the sick person, delineated a set of precepts. The theory of the 'sick role' set out by Parsons twenty-five years ago states that illness is a deviation from normal functioning which affords the sick person temporary exemption from certain social responsibilities on the grounds that he cannot be expected to look after himself or dispose of the illness through will power. As corollary to the exemption from normal duties the patient is expected to want to get well, obliged to seek competent medical help and co-operate with prescribed treatment. This construction is rooted in a view of society which defines all social positions within a set of institutionalised expectations which generate both rights and obligations.

Thus the role of the medical profession in the illness process is defined and reinforced by the ways in which doctors behave; and the universalised expectations of patients are conditioned by what they believe the doctor expects of them. This neat reciprocal arrangement is transmitted to the student physician by his teachers who are so convinced of its authenticity that they have enshrined it in codes of professional practice. A number of studies of medical education have drawn attention to the importance of learning to think and act as a doctor should and have spoken of the primary learning experience as that of socialisation into the values and practices of medicine.[6] Such writers conceive of the doctor—patient relationship as one in which technical knowledge is exercised by practitioners with 'affective neutrality' and who exercise the right to 'functional autonomy'. This means nothing less than that doctors should have no emotional involvement with the patient; will be merely applying scientific knowledge and techniques; and because of their training must always be right. Such a view is less widespread now than hitherto, but the assurance with which it was felt, not so very long ago, is well illustrated by the words of Lord Thomas Horder, Royal physician through five reigns, who said: 'Only the doctor knows what good doctoring is.'[7]

Ever since these propositions about illness and about doctors were put forward they have been the object of criticism. At an early stage Becker and colleagues[8] set out detailed evidence on the negotiative and uncertain processes of medical training from observations of student culture and behaviour. Through participant observation studies and interviews, they built up a picture of the medical school career as one where the student had to drop any ideal concept he might have had in favour of techniques which got him through exams and kept him in favour with his professors. *Boys in White* illuminated the small-scale process of the social action of medical school life [9]—what Strauss called 'status passage'—and in so doing led others to look closely at the action out of the professional role and at the realities of behaviour in medical consultations. In summing up a paper on nurse education— which he described as 'doctrinal conversion'—Fred Davis [10] captured the essence of this alternative sociological focus.

> It remains for sociology to generate models of professional socialization that are far more faithful to this picture of thinking, feeling, ever-responding and calculating *human* actors. . .models, in other words, which in their sociological richness and complexity transcend the dominant one available today—that of neutral receptive vessels into whom knowledgeable, expert members of a profession pour approved skills, attitudes and values.

It is to a selection of the studies which share Davis's concern for more 'transactional' accounts of human behaviour that attention now turns, for it is there that we shall gain some insight into the way medicine is already much modified both by its clients and by the ways doctors and nurses in particular have changed their own practices.

Illness and People

Much of the relatively short history of medical sociology has been taken up with a re-examination of the nature of illness, how individuals respond to it and the way it is resolved or coped with. In proceeding with this analysis of the position of the patient in medical care it is possible to summarise this work under headings which relate to two questions: (i) Is illness really a clearly-defined entity? (ii) How do people behave when they think they are ill?

Definitions of Illness

The 'systems' model of illness as advanced primarily by Parsons gives no real attention to the ways in which morbid conditions are defined. It is taken for granted that universal definitions exist which are shared by doctors and patients. Yet this consensus, although encouraged by that practice of medicine where all symptoms are assumed to be part of a disease entity, is clearly a mirage.

Aubrey Lewis wrote:

> Anyone who has reflected on the many definitions of health, and
> of mental health in particular, will I think, conclude that there is no
> consensus, and he will see that when moral or social values are in-
> voked there are scarcely any limits to the behaviour which might be
> called morbid.[11]

In the definition and labelling of physical illness there are historical,
cultural and economic factors involved. Fundamental to any notion of
illness is that it causes impairment of normal fulfilling of work and family
tasks and for this reason Parsons' observations have been attacked
as being ethnocentric, being defined only in terms of American
values and habits.[12] But conditions which are admissible as illness in the
US may be seen as normal or unproblematic in less technological and
medically sophisticated societies, e.g. rheumatism, migraine, or halluci-
nations.[13]

Mechanic[14] reports an interesting case of this conflict between
culture and the medical stage a particular society has reached. He des-
cribes a tribe of South American Indians, most of whom have blue
spots over their bodies which the tribesmen consider cosmetically
desirable. Indeed men who have none of these spots are marked out as
deviant and unmanly, thus losing their right to marry. American medical scientists diagnosed the blue sport to be symptom of the dietary
deficiency disease, dyschromic spirochetosis. Thus the majority were
declared sick and the deviant minority the only health ones. There is
no system of evaluating the relative rightness or goodness of trans-
cultural differences of interpretation. Whether the Indians or the
medical men have the superior explanation depends on the criteria
you choose to apply.

The situation raises important if equally thorny issues. Is it possible that the majority of a population will ever define themselves as
ill even when they have manifestly degenerated? It seems unlikely and
historical experience such as in pre-war Germany bears testimony.
Samuel Butler[15] in *Erewhon,* a cruelly ironic parody of Victorian
health and morality, illuminates the human ability to countenance and
legitimise the evil and the ridiculous as long as those in power are prepared to live with it. He depicts a fictitious land where illness is treated
as a crime, and crime as an illness. He points up the farcical nature of
many of our legal and medical beliefs through characters like Mr
Nosibor who was just getting over a bad attack of embezzlement, but

receiving visitors and condolences. Through a long and detailed description of the trial of a man in his twenties for 'persistent offences of pulmonary consumption and aggravated bronchitis', the reader witnesses a horrifying catalogue of prejudices and value judgements. It was the technique of parody which uncovered the unpleasant truth of Victorian double standards for rich and poor. Nor surprisingly, it made the establishment of the day quiver with rage. In a very different way Roger Bastide[16] was raising the same question in examining the concept of mental illness. Following a discussion of the ways in which mental illness is defined and finding them to be either normative or relativist (i.e. by comparison with some other man made standard) he asked the telling question: Can a society go mad?

Statistical prevalence has long been one of the bases of definitions of health and normality, and as these vary from society to society, there is no agreed set of interpretive rules. Sociological studies have well established how personal, social and cultural differences occur in responses to what appear to be the same symptoms. Zborowski[17] and Zola[18] have both described the different responses of Irish, Italian and American men to pain and illness, explaining these differences in terms of traditional beliefs, ethnic optimism or pessimism, societal demands of physical fitness in order to succeed and of family structure. Petrie[19] also looked at pain responses, but at the different ways individuals within a culture behave and think. Her researches led to the construction of a personality-linked continuum of 'augmenters' who amplify painful stimuli and 'reducers' who accommodate stimuli without apparent concern.

Illness, then, may be defined in one way, according to medical criteria but, in another way, the social evaluation of the importance of the condition is the significant factor in action both from patients and from doctors. Yet, as will be seen, in both cases there is a great deal of negotiation involved in the process of definition.

Illness and Behaviour

One of the most coherent criticisms of the 'sick role' theory was put forward by Mechanic,[20] who pointed out that it took no heed of what David Robinson[21] later called the process of becoming ill. Mechanic called this process 'illness behaviour' and defined it as 'the way in which given symptoms may be differentially perceived, evaluated and acted (or not acted) upon by different kinds of persons'.

People with symptoms do not automatically declare themselves ill and take to their beds, nor do they necessarily consult a doctor. As

Mechanic suggests, there is a wide range of responses which themselves are derived, for example, from experience, folk law, the need to complete tasks, or to earn money. In fact, examination of actual illness-defining behaviour makes one realise immediately that there is an enormous pool of tolerated illness in the population at any one time which has been ignored, normalised or left to develop. This submerged part of the iceberg of disease is also, as the metaphor suggests, the greater bulk of it.

Successive studies have indicated that almost everyone is experiencing symptoms of physical or mental discomfort at any given time. Wadsworth, Butterfield and Blaney[22] in their study of 2,153 adults in Bermondsey and Southwark confirmed earlier findings. Only 5 per cent of the people interviewed said they were free from symptoms or ailments of any kind. The other 95 per cent reported complaints occurring during the two weeks prior to the interview. Nineteen per cent of these took no action and 76 per cent were taking action of various kinds. Of the total survey population the investigators, using their own criteria, considered that over half needed further investigation which would possibly lead to medical treatment.

Mental illness, though notoriously difficult to define, also exists in far larger quantities than that which is reported to doctors. One estimate, using World Health Organisation criteria, put the level of psychiatric illness at more than half of the population.[23] More restrained definitions employed by psychiatrists at the Maudsley Hospital[24] put the figure of emotionally disturbed people at about one in eight. Yet it is well known that people who are disturbed rarely take their condition to the doctor except when disguised as part of a more 'acceptable' physical complaint. Resulting from this reluctance, there is again a substantial submerged iceberg.

If a visit to the general practitioner is not the first line of defence, what action normally follows the emergence of symptoms? In fact there is no simple answer to this question. People respond to symptoms mainly as a way of coping with them until they recede and vanish, or reach a threshold of tolerance where the condition becomes threatening in some way. Typically, the first line of defence for all but the immediately serious and traumatic is self-medication. Dunnell and Cartwright[25] found that 41 per cent of their national sample had taken pain killers during the preceding fortnight, 14 per cent indigestion remedies, 14 per cent skin ointments or antiseptics; 13 per cent throat or cough remedies, and many others including gargles, alcohol, embrocation, rejuvenators and suppositories.

Over-the-counter sales of pharmaceutical and other preparations are big business. Brian Abel-Smith,[26] in examining the ethics and economics of the drug industry, comments:

> Throughout the world patients also buy a wide range of medicines without a medical prescription. In the United States, the average citizen spent $21.52 for prescribed drugs and $14.14 for other drugs and sundries in 1971. In more developed countries, aspirin and its derivatives, vitamin preparations, tonics and laxatives represent substantial shares of the non-prescription drug market. In many developing countries people incur heavy expenditure on traditional herbal remedies.

In Britain the bill for drugs prescribed by general practitioners came to £272 million in 1974, whilst the amount spent on over-the-counter medicines was approximately £95 million, or one-third of the amount spent on NHS prescriptions. The 1973 Family Expenditure Survey reports that in a sample two-week period 58 per cent of households bought some kind of over-the-counter medicines (including dressings). The average amount per week for each household was 20 pence.[27] In interpreting these figures it should be remembered that the most expensive drugs are not available without prescription and thus the number of *occasions* on which self-prescribed medication was taken may well rival those prescribed by doctors.

In addition to the now conventional consumption of drugs to assuage symptoms there remains a substantial amount of traditional healing practices in common use. In Africa there is syncretisation of modern scientific medicine with magical and folk remedies.[28] Sociologists and anthropologists have given much more attention to this predictable phenomenon, than to its counterpart in developed societies. None the less Coe,[29] in reviewing the still slender American literature, demonstrates the variety and magnitude of non-medical approaches to illness ranging from homeopathy to full-blown magical rituals. In teasing out the magical elements in modern medicine Tina Carmeli[30] heightens our awareness of the important place metaphysical beliefs and symbolic rituals have in the whole gamut of 'getting well' behaviour.

Successors to the Carbolic Smoke Ball are to be found widely advertised in Sunday newspapers and periodicals. Miracle cures appear to continue to thrive despite the Trades Descriptions Act; but there is also a growth in consultation with practitioners of non-medical healing like osteopaths, chiropractors and acupuncturists. Hard information about the actual size of this market and the number of practitioners is hard to come by. Hewitt and Wood[31] produced figures in 1975 of some categories of heterodox practitioners who are registered with the semi-official bodies which represent them. There were 61 acupuncturists, 167 naturopaths, 116 homeopaths (medically qualified), 75 chiropractors, 296 registered osteopaths and 60 non-registered. They go on to suggest that 'On available evidence it would seem that something like two hundred thousand people consult an osteopath or chiropractor during the course of a year'. Later estimates suggest that both the number of practitioners and the number of people who consult them is much under-estimated by these figures. None the less they indicate a very substantial field of healing activity outside of orthodox allopathic medicine.

In a similar way, self-care in illness and disability has in recent years become a much more organised affair. Mutual self-care groups exist for many specific conditions, like Alcoholics Anonymous, Weight Watchers, British Diabetics Association, The Phobics Society, Royal National Institute for the Blind and hundreds of others which exist to help sufferers cope better alone, by drawing on the experience of others. David Robinson[32] has pointed out that many of these groups, far from establishing a separation from medicine, become extensions of prescribed medical régimes and engage medical advisers to formulate policy. His argument is convincing in some cases and especially when the condition is mainly physiological. However, within this range there are many groups and movements which have adopted homeopathic and naturopathic approaches based on the rejection of orthodox medicine.

For some sufferers these and other unorthodox healers are the last resort after medical failure, as Cobb[33] has shown for cancer cases. Yet for many they are positive commitments to the kind of alternative medical system prescribed by Illich.[34] Ideologically they represent the distant polarity from modern medicine, adopting healthiness as a base for living. Michael Wilson's book *Health is for People*[35] deserves attention for its sensitive and passionate exposition of the healthy non-medical life. In it he explains the nature of health in many ways, but two of them put his case: 'There is no way to health through the cure of illness.' 'Health is not for the rich to give to the poor. Health is a quality of life they make together.'

Those in the natural health movement view orthodox medical practices as health-polluting and monopolising and thus have no or only minimal contact with it.[36] Others hesitate about seeking the aid of a physician for diverse reasons. The literature has come to term this as 'patient delay'. Early studies adopted the Parsonian paradigm of behaviour and thus tried to explain why sick people should behave in apparently irrational ways. As a result enquiries like Goldsen's[37] on cancer patients defined 'delayers' as those who waited more than three months before seeking a doctor, and who were more likely to be rural residents and to have lower levels of income, occupation and education than non-delayers. This type of classificatory approach has given way to studies of the social, psychological and economic reasons for non-consultation, focusing on accounts of actual behaviour and analysis of the thinking which gave rise to the actions. Irving Zola[38] identified five 'triggers' in patients' decisions to seek (or not to seek) medical care, summarised as Interpersonal Crisis, Social Interference, The Presence of Sanctions, Perceived Threat, and Nature and Quality of the Symptoms. Mechanic[39] set out an even more elaborate scheme based on ten key variables which precipitate doctor consultation. These and other studies have centred on closer analysis of individual behaviour rather than on establishing the explanatory potency of socio-demographic factors. This type of work has led to recent and current small-scale studies which seek to uncover the meaning of common-sense and everyday life as it impinges on illness and illness on it. Una Maclean's[40] study of 32 heart attack patients has led her to challenge the medical belief that infarction is an instantaneous and dramatic event and that patient delay is therefore frequently an inappropriate and wrong-headed label. Her evidence, based upon detailed reconstructions by coronary patients, indicates that the pains were frequently passed off as indigestion and not of the sort which produce paroxysms of pain.

Extended attention has been given to the way people think and behave prior to going to see the doctor because although no one clear simple picture emerges, it is material to the argument that patients have a great deal more control over illness situations than is commonly thought. The choice about whether to seek medical attention or not is a real if problematic one for most people. And if the evidence is to be believed, very few consult without due thought and consideration about the significance of the symptoms to them nor without some clear idea as to what they want from seeing the doctor. Attending a surgery is therefore the culmination of one process and the beginning of another; for, as the author wrote once before:

the individual must first perceive his condition, then evaluate its seriousness. Given that these two processes have been gone through and he finds it needful of professional attention, he must present his problem to an appropriate agency and be sufficiently articulate to allow proper diagnosis.[41]

Thus having mapped out the area of illness-defining behaviour and noted that it encompasses the majority of symptoms without medical aid, it is essential to look at the way illnesses referred to a physician are handled by both parties.

The Consultation Process

In his performance of the classic sketch 'The Blood Donor', Tony Hancock prefaces the business of giving blood with a string of pleasantries that verge on the obsequious. Having had a pin-prick test taken and in full readiness for his tea and biscuit, he is alarmed to find a whole pint of his blood is required. The doctor says that what he has given is 'only a smear', to which Hancock retorts, 'It may be a smear to you, mate, but it's life and death to some poor devil.' Although the circumstances are peculiar, the scene represents an important dilemma in all doctor—patient relationships. The consultation process is commonly accepted as one in which the deferential patient acts as a passive receiver. In reality the deference is frequently only the acting out of a traditional role. Indeed by his very presence there the patient has, at least in general terms, already decided what he wants out of the encounter and has chosen to consult his doctor in the belief that his needs will be appropriately supplied.

In the structural-functionalist model the patient behaves according to expectations which are socially agreed and upon which the physician has come to rely. He therefore projects them on to the patient. There can be no doubt that medical practitioners do frequently continue to hold to the views of doctors' and patients' roles set out in this model and still taught in medical schools. But increasingly this sort of behaviour only serves to heighten the conflict of which Freidson[42] has spoken, rather than to perpetuate the controlled interchange which the medical student was also taught to expect. Freidson commented: 'the separate worlds of experience and reference of the layman and the professional worker are always in potential conflict with each other.'

Evidence from medical sociological studies is tantalisingly conflicting. Large social surveys are almost unanimous in telling us that patient satisfaction with doctors is very high. Smaller-scale studies are equally in agreement that doctor—patient interactions are problematic and conflict-ridden. Therefore to look at a small selection of this work is necessary if the argument is to be advanced a step further. This examination will be mainly confined to studies of general practice because it deals with the vast majority of physician-treated illness and because the environment of the hospital places peculiar constraints on the ability of patients to manage their contacts with health professionals of all types.[43]

Ann Cartwright's study of 1,397 patients and their 422 general practitioners is one of the major contributions to this area of interest.[44] From her respondents only 4 per cent of patients were thoroughly critical of their doctors, all the rest finding complimentary and understanding things to say about him. Eighteen per cent said he was friendly and approachable, 24 per cent thoughtful, considerate, understanding or sympathetic, 19 per cent that he visited promptly and without grumbling, 12 per cent thorough or conscientious. There were criticisms of course. Yet, by contrast, only 5 per cent felt he did not always listen, 5 per cent criticised his manner, 2 per cent thought he did not go into things properly and 3 per cent thought he gave unsatisfactory care. At the end of the book she concludes:

> If a plebiscite was held on whether patients wished to retain the general practitioner service or change to a system in which front-line medical care was based on specialists and hospitals, there is little doubt that the result would be overwhelmingly in favour of the present arrangement. But behind the satisfaction of most patients there lies an uncritical acceptance and lack of discrimination which is conducive to stagnation and apathy.

Patient satisfaction surveys in hospitals reinforce the image that is retained of the Cartwright study, giving a sense that all but the disputatious minority are contented with the medical care that they get.[45] Even the very latest gargantuan cross-national study lends its massive statistical weight to this view. Based on interviews with an unprecedented 47,000 people in twelve study areas spread over seven countries, the editors conclude that satisfaction with physician contact is high everywhere, irrespective of the nature of the health systems. Only 5 per cent of the interviewees said they were dissatisfied.[46]

It appears inevitable that social surveys, which are primarily about consultations and the medical conditions which gave rise to them, will provide reassuring conclusions when the evaluative questions are tacked on at the end. What is interesting is the way such studies produce such a watertight view of the situation. In the quotation above there is reference to patient apathy and passiveness. In fact she wrote, 'Most doctors agreed that a good general practitioner could train his patients not to make unnecessary or unreasonable demands on him and two-fifths of all consultations, 57 per cent of follow-ups and 64 per cent of home visits were felt, by the patient, to have been initiated by the doctor.' Raphael writes in much the same terms as did Cartwright[47] in an earlier study of hospital care, where lack of information was the main cause of anxiety. It is indeed true that official complaints against the GP and hospital services are few, but as will be observed later on, these represent only the tip of another iceberg of which American surveyors like Koos[48] and Freidson[49] have given forewarning.

Smaller-scale studies offer an alternative view, Julius Roth's participant-observation study of TB patients in hospital[50] and Fred Davis's account of how families cope with the situation where a child contracts polio[51] have provided models for other researchers. In the case of the TB patient, the search for information upon which a scale of progress and time-tabling can be constructed is a dominant theme. Roth shows how the sick person is starved of the facts and the progress reports he needs, and therefore resorts to elaborate consultations with other patients so as to build up from that lay referral system a set of expectations about the time of recovery and the benchmarks along the way. Davis also gives much attention to the negotiation which goes on between doctors and patients. In the nature of the polio disease there is little basis for medical prediction, yet there is a great hunger for information which is mainly denied.

The reciprocity in the doctor—patient relationship implied by the surveys of patient satisfaction begins to look very flimsy when examined at close quarters. Bloor and Horobin[52] suggest that fundamen-mentally the relationship is one of conflict rooted in the expectations that doctors have of patients, so clearly expressed by Cartwright. Doctors expect patients to use their own judgement about when it is appropriate to seek medical advice; but later expect them to defer to superior judgement when undergoing medical treatment. On the one hand, patients are assumed to be their own diagnosticians (as indeed they must be to present their symptoms in the first place) but then accept the professional view however much it may differ from their own assessment. Lee and Gunawardena[53] make a similar point about the way in which people who present themselves at Accident and Emergency departments not only self-diagnose but decide positively against going to the GP. This way of getting primary medical care is often considered an abuse of the hospital service, but it can also be seen as well-calculated patient behaviour.

This 'double-bind' of patient independence and professional control produces no problems at all for some patients who have learned to accept such paradoxes as normal. But for a few it produces disagreements which result in the patient seeking a new GP—a theoretically possible but difficult procedure under the NHS. More commonly patients who disagree take matters into their own hands outside of the consulting room. As we have already seen, lay and unorthodox advice is sought and acted upon and this frequently leads to the disregarding of medically prescribed treatment régimes.[54] But predictably no single mode of behaviour forms the response to dissonant interpretations of symptoms. The range extends from complete acquiescence to outright rejection. Yet whenever differences do occur which the patient finds unacceptable, he may adopt a number of available strategies for re-negotiating previous diagnoses and treatments.

As Bloor and Horobin point out, most consultations are only one of a series and thus harmony may emerge over time as each encounter brings doctor and patient closer to an understanding. Indeed the dialogue over the interpretation of each set of symptoms might be seen as individual experience to which expectations of the doctor are attached, rather than there being a set of generalised expectations for all situations. Robinson provides a number of very clear examples of the special requirements patients attach to conditions and situations in his study of fourteen families in South Wales who recorded health diaries for him.[55] Reading these accounts, one is made acutely aware of illness as a process and a process which has dramaturgical forms and properties. Following through accounts of illness episodes, it becomes clear that they have dialogue, form and even plot. The negotiation between the central actor—the symptomatic person—and his significant others (his family, friends and acquaintances) is in itself drama.[56]

In their study of the consultation process in general practice, Stimson and Webb placed major emphasis on the way this process is managed as a social activity.[57] And in order to see the face-to-face contact within the context of the whole process, they also paid attention to what, for the patient, goes on before and after the consultation. Once the often elaborately formed decision to consult has been made it leads to more or less conscious planning of the next stages.

Anticipating the encounter may begin long before the person is seated in the waiting room. It is, in fact, difficult to divorce this anticipation from the decision-making involved in perceiving a problem as an appropriate one for the doctor's attention. . . This anticipatory period may also include a mental construction of the encounter in terms of how such consultations are usually conducted, how events might proceed in this instance, and the possible outcome and the ways of achieving certain desired ends. Such a construction may also involve the person in considering the likely and probable reactions of the doctor. The person then plans what to say if the doctor follows one course rather than another. For instance, one woman whose doctor had earned the nickname 'Two-minute Todd' reflecting the supposed speed with which he conducted his consultations, intended to try to prolong the encounter in order to clarify her problem and was planning ways of counteracting her expected dismissal by the doctor.

However the consultation goes, and whatever the outcome, it only forms part of the ongoing drama of the illness episode. Most consultations result in a prescription. The usefulness of the drugs is assessed and the medicine is taken or rejected according to experience, prejudice and whim. The consultation is also evaluated against previous expectations. Eighty-three per cent had had an expected outcome and thus were able to weigh it up in these terms. Dissatisfied and satisfied patients tend to talk out the encounter in order to legitimise the experience and to establish expectations of what should follow with relatives and friends. Just to underscore the essentially social nature of the exercise, the study shows how each patient's account of the consultation depicts him as the hero. The dramaturgical nature of the process is thus drawn out and the meeting of doctor and patient is placed in the context of human biographies rather than viewed within the narrow confines of the consulting room.

Consumerism, Deference and the Professions

A latent kind of consumerism has already been discussed. It is the manner in which patients exercise varying degrees of control over the way their illnesses are managed. If this established pattern is placed in a context of changing relationships between customers and clients on the one hand and retailers and service providers on the other, then it is likely that a more equal and participative arrangement will emerge. But before going on to look at the consumer movement, it is worth taking a look at the notion of deference.

Reference has already been made to the tacit agreement in society at large about the deferential nature of the patient role. It remains largely

unchallenged because it underpins many of the hierarchical relationships that continue in modern Britain. The nature of class relations has
undoubtedly changed even since the war, but there is still a substantial
residue of behaviour ranging from the ingratiating to acquiescence in
the 'establishment' view. Sociologists and political scientists have done
little to dispel the view that deference is a continuing part of, in particular, working-class life in the workplace, in voting behaviour, in
consumer habits and in all areas of authority, despite some of their own
findings to the contrary.[58]

Howard Newby[59] has examined the literature on deference and feels
that it fails to come to terms with the many discrepancies in expected
and real situations because it does not distinguish clearly enough between behaviour, attitudes and socially held beliefs. Thus deferential
behaviour should not be taken as confirmation of a deferential attitude.
It may merely be a useful mode of achieving some desirable end like
getting a sick note or time off work to go to a wedding. This is the
mode of behaviour that Goffman[60] calls 'impression management' and
one which is used when people are 'on stage'. The metaphor of social
drama is again employed here and the term 'on stage' refers to, say, the
behaviour of a butler when talking with his employer and who then
goes 'off stage' below stairs.

A good deal of deferential behaviour is ritualised and habitual like
the soldier's salute and the addressing of customers in shops as 'madam'
and 'sir'. Consequently it cannot be used as a reasonable guide to the
attitudes it represents. If deference is to be meaningful the behaviour
must faithfully represent an attitude and not just be a piece of impression management. Therefore, Newby suggests that 'real' deference
occurs only where there is a congruence of behaviour and attitudes,
but that deferential *behaviour* which denies the underlying attitude is
calculative and thus in essence non-deferential.

In relations between the providers and consumers of services there
has been a clear shift in behaviour in recent years. There is more assertiveness and less passivity. Consumerism has grown up in America and
Western Europe in the past decade manifesting itself in nation-wide
organisations like the Consumers' Association in Britain and the Ralph
Nader organisations in the US. Their first concerns were with the re-
establishment of the buyers' rights in relation to manufactured goods,
attention later moving to the quality of service provided by retailers
and maintenance firms. Nader led a crusade against the power of com-
mercial interests, whilst in Britain the less emotive response was more
directed at ensuring those merchantable qualities and rights which

frequently existed in the Sale of Goods Act 1893, but were submerged by time and practice. By the mid-seventies consumer-protecting legislation had become enormous, as had the machinery for its enforcement, though not fully operational to achieve the objectives of the legislation.

Organisations for the better informing and better representation of the 'ordinary' consumer have grown up in many fields of activity. As well as the bodies which advise on the quality of goods and services offered for sale, there is an impressive number of agencies which offer the same service for such 'groups' as alcoholics, the mentally ill, those receiving social security, the single-parent family, the homeless, the old, the physically disabled and the politically oppressed. Not all of the groups which provide this sort of advice and support are new, but even those which have been in the field a long time (Age Concern in its former guise as the National Old People's Welfare Council, the Councils for Voluntary Service, MIND as its other self The National Association for Mental Health, serve as good examples) have newly taken on the clear role of social advocate and representative—a theme developed in a less sanguine manner by Ham in his analysis of consumer groups in the NHS.[61]

Citizens Advice Bureaux, Housing Advice Centres, Claimants Union stalls, Pregnancy Advisory Service and Family Planning clinics, Legal Advice Centres, CPAG, and Shelter offices are all familiar sources of information on a national scale. Moreover these bodies will frequently help complainants to lodge their complaint and in some cases act as spokesman and intermediary. It is therefore possible to make a case for the emergence of consumerism as a force to be reckoned with. Yet its main thrust has been confined to consumer durables and related activities. Now this emphasis is also to be found in bodies which represent the claims of the poor, sick and inarticulate to administrations and bureaucracies.

Whilst it might be claimed that professional services have remained relatively free of informed intermediaries, in fact lawyers, doctors, accountants, architects, chartered engineers and academics have all received adverse media coverage and assaults of a kind of late.[62] But the knowledge gap and the elaborate self-regulatory defensive mechanisms have so far held client retaliation at arm's length. None the less it could be advanced that consumer pressure groups of an effective and radical kind are beginning to emerge as a challenge to these professions. Indeed, in some cases the professions have turned on themselves as in the case of community legal advice centres and in the recent questioning by solicitors and barristers of their practices. Yet, self-interest groups by consumers are not much in evidence. Indeed one of the salutary facts about the consumers of professional services is that whilst they might complain bitterly (or give praise) about the treatment they receive it is usually done in private. There appears to be little which binds such complainants together, partly perhaps because once they have survived a particular series of traumatic events they have neither the desire nor the energy to relive them with little prospect of recompense. In addition, the professions' reputation for closing ranks and deflecting complaints, whether well-founded or not, may itself act as a deterrent.

In consequence, the Patients' Association has been made up mainly of those who have had the necessary stamina and the knowledge to fight for others. In the context of this paper what is important about the Patients' Association has been its refusal to play the conventional role of layman. The officers and staff have ensured that they are well-informed on medical matters, though not medically trained. Their strength in argument with the health professions is the combination of this knowledge with a refusal to accept that doctors necessarily know best. Even the pretence of deference is stripped away and discussion about complaints is grounded in a clear view of what is humane and tolerable, regardless of the technical explanations.

The Patients' Association is not new, though until reorganisation of the NHS in 1974 it was the only national organisation of its type. With the coming of Community Health Councils in the new NHS the Association considered closing down in the belief that the CHCs would do their job. In fact CHCs were specifically directed away from handling complaints. The reality, though, is that whilst CHCs do deal with a lot of complaints the Patients' Association still finds a role for itself in campaigning, providing information and picking up those complaints which some CHCs fail to hear about or carry through.

Until 1974 there was very little in the way of organised support for the unsatisfied consumer of health and medical services. But aware of the growth of participation at all levels of organisations, the Conservative government had introduced specific and separate consumer representation for the first time. If CHCs are not the vehicle for laying to rest the traditional view of the ever-deferential layman, they do appear—at least to this writer—to be the main route through which a gradual transformation of the status of the patient is likely to materialise.

Power to the Patient?

This essay has attempted to indicate the mythical status of much that is written about the total subservience and acquiescence of patients, particularly in relation to the GP with whom they have the great majority of contacts. In so doing it is not claimed that 'client control' is now the norm, for this is clearly not the case. But the picture of unrelieved medical dominance is challenged in so far as doctors increasingly take account of rising patient expectations based on greater knowledge and the public view of what the NHS has to offer.[63] Note has also been made of an emergent challenge to the hold that professionals of all sorts have over their territories. The evidence for their dominance is still impressively strong,[64] but there are good reasons for believing that as in other fields the ideology of consumerism is increasing in medicine. This paper has also attempted to draw out the amount of negotiability which already commonly exists in doctor—patient relationships. Even acknowledging the relative ignorance patients have of medical terms[65] and the continuing class gradient in consultation time[66] and quality of care,[67] there are strong grounds for believing that trends in patient behaviour will force, perhaps already have forced, doctors to re-assess their own attitudes and ways of conducting themselves.[68]

Some indications can be offered of this modification of medical attitudes and behaviour, though not all in the direction which the public would have wished. For one thing, although there has been a steady flow into general practice from hospital medicine since the 'GPs' charter' of the mid-sixties came to fruition, it has not been matched with an equal commitment to full clinical duties. Although GPs are contracted with the NHS to provide 24-hour cover for seven days a week, in reality, and in some ways not unreasonably, many are now prepared to pay out of their own pockets for deputising services to cover their night and week-end responsibilities. More surprisingly, perhaps, even in city areas where large group practices exist which could more easily provide rota arrangements, it is increasingly common for GPs to contract into a deputising scheme. Whilst such schemes are not necessarily the best ways of meeting the need, they do relieve general practitioners from a burden of round-the-clock responsibility which many now believe to be excessive. Expectations of GPs have been enormously high and one aspect of the current fluid situation may be the downward revision of what the consumer demands and expects of his doctor.

Indeed, it might be speculated that withdrawal from clinical work into other more rewarding fields appears to be one of the hallmarks of present-day medicine. The author's current research on the careers of medical graduates suggests that many doctors with established careers—and therefore established expectations—find the contemporary medical scene either too confusing or too threatening. One of the responses to the feeling that medicine is in decline and that doctors are losing their traditional autonomy is to work less and play more or spend more time with the family. Another is to become involved in medical politics, perhaps in order to retrieve some of the lost autonomy.

In the hospital sphere there are similar movements. As both Elston and Dimmock[69] point out, the growth of bargaining power amongst health workers in hospitals has influenced relationships between doctors and their non-medical colleagues. For some it has become an opportunity to work more effectively in multi-disciplinary teams. But change is not universally accepted and leads to resentment or frustration in some quarters. Symptomatic of these feelings have been their campaigns for more money and the juniors and their seniors have both resorted in an unparalleled way to strike behaviour previously condemned as unprofessional.

Yet, though the medical profession may have become more vociferous of late it may also have to live increasingly with assaults on its own domain as medicine becomes more publicly accountable. For instance, whilst in their report the Davies Committee on Hospital Complaints Procedure[70] wrote: 'At the moment, between 8,000 and 9,000 written complaints made by patients or on their behalf are investigated each year by hospital authorities in England and Wales, which represents a fraction of 1 per cent of the annual total of in-patients,' an enquiry they commissioned also showed that approximately 4 per cent of patients interviewed after discharge had made oral complaints or suggestions for improvements during the course of their stay. Complaints against GPs are equally infrequent though they must be made either direct to the doctor or to the little-known Family Practitioner Committees. Formal procedures for both have existed for some years, but they require confidence, articulacy and staying power. Moreover the procedures, which are ill-publicised, are all effectively 'internal' in that they are conducted by those who are directly or indirectly responsible for the services concerned.

Consideration of the Davies Committee Report has been long delayed, but recently resulted in DHSS issuing a draft circular on a new Complaints Procedure, to be implemented in 1977. The outcome of the discussions is still awaited, but the prospect is that health workers of all sorts and doctors in particular will become much more accountable to their patients, and that Community Health Councils may come to play an important part in monitoring the system. This will greatly extended their current practice of assisting complainants in informal ways. In addition, the Secretary of State in February 1976 invited the Select Committee on the Parliamentary Commissioner for Administration (who is also the Health Commissioner) to review the arrangements for the *independent investigation* of complaints which arise in hospitals. This review is to deal with procedures over and above the new Complaints Procedure; so it can reasonably be expected that together they will introduce a complaints machinery which will serve to radically open up discussion about quality of service. The complaints issue tends to crystallise the differences of view between those who provide medical services and those who receive them. But the discussion about creating more equality between the parties is concerned with redefining the relationship and the processes that the medical enterprise comprises. It is also concerned with a re-examination of the outcomes which people want from health care. Medical education continues to transmit to student doctors traditional views about patient expectations, which some of the students and some of their educators have themselves begun to question. This questioning must of necessity go further into the established profession as the pressure for patient involvement and consultation about what is to be done *for* him rather than *to* him, increases.

Partly as a result of this official widening in medicine's public accountability, it is suggested that a new phase in the involvement of patients will begin. But it follows close on the heels of another. Community Health Councils were established to represent the patient and in varying degree have begun to do that. There is a wide range of performance, as Hallas shows,[71] but a sufficient number of CHCs have made their mark for there to be confidence in their future ability to raise the level of debate in a way which will make doctors, nurses and administrators revise their view of current unsatisfactory services and their priorities for the use of resources.[72] The common experience of CHCs is accumulating in an impressive way, so that the weak are learning from the strong. There will, of course, remain a residue of Councils which are basically ineffective, but one can only be impressed by the commitment and involvement that characterises much of the CHC world. Their critics continue to point to the lack of formal powers, but some commentators[73] have seen this as a positive advantage to be exploited. Additional CHC involvement with the consumer of health care in the context of a more open system could provide for the first time a corporate expression of the individual voices previously muffled by the formality of doctor—patient consultations. People who consult doctors do not go blindly or without some notion of their purpose. Nor are they incapable of judging what they think good and bad medicine might be. Therefore, without placing undue faith and optimism on the impact of CHCs, they can be seen to represent a crucial stage in the emergence of participative medicine and one which could prove to be a climacteric.

Whether this patient involvement is an expression of consumerism or not is perhaps a semantic debate. Certainly it has every appearance of being part of that movement. Margaret Stacey has expressed doubts about patient consumerism on the grounds that the patient is viewed as more of a 'work object' than as a 'consumer'.[74] However this analysis only defines past and, to a lesser extent, current practices, for if the basis of the relationship can be democratised the patient will cease to have the status of object and become a participant. What is clear is that for sociological analysis there is as yet no appropriate term to describe the patient as 'social actor'. The phrase 'patient as partner, but also as work object' is offered but must necessarily be unusable except as a reminder that new situations are emergent that require not only new attitudes but new language.

Patient demands for participation and their increasing, if modest, use of formal machinery to achieve desired ends along with greater use of personal strategies has already made its mark on the medical world. Yet it might be argued that if participation is to take on a real meaning, participant patients, CHCs and other 'consumer' bodies will need to involve themselves further in the politics of health care. If the bodies which represent those who receive health care take their tasks at all seriously, then they must advance a more participative form of medicine. The base for this development is long established in the manipulative devices which patients have employed beneath the flimsy guise of deferent behaviour. In a society with high levels of education and mass media communication it is possible for the ordinary citizen to learn much about the professional preserves of specialist knowledge. Even when he does not have matching knowledge he has become increasingly aware of a network of information-providers at his disposal. The concept of layman is being remodelled so that it incorporates the ability to ask intelligent questions and to expect intelligent and intelligible answers.

In all this excavation of the consumer's emergent identity, the profession's own responses should not be ignored. Participative rights will not be handed out on a plate by doctors or nurses or administrators. They will all fight to preserve their own territories and in so doing slow up the process. Consumers will need to heed the consequences of their assertiveness on the professionals, just as the professionals already have to face a more sophisticated audience for their work. None the less, if the present trend continues, patients will no longer be prepared to accept Shaw's diagnosis that all professions are conspiracies against the laity.

Notes

1. A. M. Carr-Saunders and P. A. Wilson, *The Professions,* Oxford University Press, Oxford, 1933.
2. Everett C. Hughes, *Men and their Work,* Free Press, Glencoe, Illinois, 1958.
3. Talcott Parsons, *The Social System,* Free Press, Glencoe, Illinois, 1951; W. J. Goode, 'Community Within a Community: The Professions', *American Sociological Review,* Vol. 22, April 1957, pp.194-208; Samuel W. Bloom, 'The Process of Becoming a Physician', *The Annals of the American Academy of Political and Social Science,* Vol. 346, March 1963, pp.77-87; R. Hall, 'Professionalization and Bureaucratization', *American Sociological Review,* Vol. 33, February 1968, pp.92-104; Eliot Freidson, *Profession of Medicine: A Study of the Sociology of Applied Knowledge,* Dodd Mead, New York, 1970; Eliot Freidson, *Professional Dominance: The Social Structure of Medical Care,* Atherton Press, New York, 1970; Irving K. Zola, 'Medicine as an Institution of Social Control', *Sociological Review,* 20, 3, November 1972; Ivan Illich, *Medical Nemesis: The Expropriation of Health,* Calder and Boyars, London, 1975. Literature on the professions has moved a long way from the early studies which tended to describe in detail the conventionally accepted view. During the past decade or so commentators have concentrated more on the value systems of professions, their exclusionist élitist policies and the nature of their relationships with clients and government. The studies cited here represent a cross-cut of the available studies in a chronological sequence which is also one of increasing criticism.
4. Talcott Parsons, op. cit., 1951.
5. Robert K. Merton *et al. The Student Physician,* Harvard University Press, Cambridge, Massachusetts, 1957.
6. This view of medical education as the learning of a body of knowledge and socialisation into the attitudes and behaviour appropriate to doctors is well illustrated in H. I. Leif and R. Fox, 'The Medical Student's Training for Detached Concern' in H. I. Leif *et al* (eds.), *The Psychological Base of Medical Practice,* Harper and Row, New York, 1964.
7. L. Cowan and M. Cowan (compilers), *The Wit of Medicine,* Leslie Frewin, London, 1972, p.22.
8. H. S. Becker *et al. Boys in White, Student Culture in the Medical School,* University of Chicago Press, Chicago, 1961.
9. Anselm L. Strauss, *Mirrors and Masks,* Free Press, Glencoe, Illinois, 1959.
10. Fred Davis, 'Professional Socialization as Subjective Experience: the Process of Doctrinal Conversion among student nurses' in H. S. Becker *et al* (eds.), *Institutions and the Person,* Aldine, Chicago, 1968, and reproduced in C. Cox and A. Meade (eds.), *A Sociology of Medical Practice,* Collier-Macmillan, London, 1975, p.130.
11. Aubrey Lewis, 'Medicine and the Affections of the Mind', *British Medical Journal,* 2, pp.1549-57, 1963.

12. The first systematic writing on the 'sick role' was based exclusively on American patterns of behaviour. A good summary of the deficiencies of this literature is contained in J. R. Butler, 'Illness and the Sick Role: An Evaluation in Three Communities', *British Journal of Sociology*, Vol. 21, 3, September 1970.

13. For example, S. Schulman and A. M. Smith, 'The Concept of Health Among Spanish Speaking Villagers of New Mexico and Colorado', *Journal of Health and Social Behaviour*, 4, Winter 1963, pp.226-45; L. Saunders, *Cultural Difference and Medical Care*, Russell Sage, New York, 1954.

14. David Mechanic, *Medical Sociology, A Selective View*, Free Press, Glencoe, Illinois, 1968.

15. Samuel Butler, *Erewhon*, Penguin Books, Harmondsworth, 1970 (First published 1872).

16. Roger Bastide addresses this question in a chapter called 'Prolegomena to a Sociology of Mental Disorder' in *The Sociology of Mental Disorder*, Routledge and Kegan Paul, London, 1972.

17. M. Zborowski, 'Cultural Components in Responses to Pain', *Journal of Social Issues*, 8, 16, 1952.

18. Irving K. Zola, 'Culture and Symptoms: An Analysis of Patients Presenting Complaints', *American Sociological Review*, 31, 5, 1960, pp.615-30.

19. A. Petrie, *Individuality in Pain and Suffering*, University of Chicago Press, Chicago, 1967.

20. David Mechanic, 'The Concept of Illness Behaviour', *Journal of Chronic Diseases*, 15, 1961, p.189.

21. David Robinson, *The Process of Becoming Ill*, Routledge and Kegan Paul, London, 1971.

22. M. E. J. Wadsworth, W. J. H. Butterfield and R. Blaney, *Health and Sickness: The Choice of Treatment*, Tavistock, London, 1971.

23. W. I. N. Kessel, 'The Psychiatric Morbidity in a London General Practice', *British Journal of Social and Preventive Medicine*, 14, 16, 1960.

24. M. Shepherd *et al.*, *Psychiatric Illness in General Practice*, Oxford University Press, London, 1966.

25. Karen Dunnell and Ann Cartwright, *Medicine Takers, Prescribers and Hoarders*, Routledge and Kegan Paul, London, 1972.

26. Brian Abel-Smith, *Value for Money in Health Services*, Heinemann, London, 1976, p.77.

27. The author is indebted to Karen Dunnell of the Office of Population and Censuses for providing this information.

28. Una Maclean, *Magical Medicine, A Nigerian Case Study*, Allen Lane, Penguin Press, London, 1973.

29. Rodney Coe, *Sociology of Medicine*, McGraw-Hill, New York, 1970.

30. T. Carmeli, 'Magical Elements of Orthodox Medicine', paper presented at British Sociological Association Annual Conference, Manchester, April 1976.

31. D. Hewitt and P. H. N. Wood, 'Heterodox Practitioners and the Availability of Specialist Advice', *Rheumatology and Rehabilitation*, 14, 191, 1975. Malcolm Hainsworth, University of Hull, from his own researches on heterodox practitioners has suggested to the author that the Hewitt and Woods estimates are far smaller than the actual numbers of both practitioners and clients, as many practitioners are not registered with even the semi-official bodies and thus their clients are also overlooked. For example he estimates that there are twice as many non-registered osteopaths and 20 per cent more chiropractors than the article indicates.

32. David Robinson, 'Mutual Self-Care and the (De-) Medcalisation of Life —

a brief note', paper presented at British Sociological Association Conference, Manchester, April 1976.

33. B. Cobb, 'Why Do Patients De-tour to Quacks?', in E. G. Jaco (ed.), *Patients, Physicians and Illness,* Free Press, New York, 1958.

34. Ivan Illich, op. cit., 1975.

35. Michael Wilson, *Health is For People,* Darton, Longman and Todd, London, 1975.

36. Julius Roth, *The Natural Health Movement in the USA,* Final Report, National Institutes of Health Research Grant HS 00564, Davis, California, November 1972.

37. R. K. Goldsen *et al.,* 'Some factors related to Patient Delay in Seeking Diagnosis for Cancer Symptoms', *Cancer,* 10, 1, January-February 1957.

38. Irving K. Zola, 'Illness Behaviour of the Working Class' in A Shostak, and W. Gomberg (eds.), *Blue Collar World: Studies of the American Worker,* Prentice-Hall, Englewood Cliffs, New Jersey, 1964.

39. David Mechanic, op. cit., 1968.

40. Una Maclean, 'Patient Delay: Some Observations on Medical Claims to Certainty', *The Lancet,* 23, 5 July 1975.

41. Malcolm L. Johnson, 'Self-Perception of Need Amongst the Elderly: An Analysis of Illness Behaviour', *Sociological Review,* Vol. 20, No. 4, November 1972.

42. Eliot Freidson, *Patients' Views of Medical Practice,* Russell Sage, New York, 1961.

43. The hospital as a social institution is greatly geared to the needs of staff and the routine practices which they adopt. Patients are only temporary residents (as a rule) of hospitals and their transient status as members of the community makes influencing its total culture difficult. Thus patients' areas of negotiation are limited. See A. L. Strauss *et al., Psychiatric Ideologies and Institutions,* Free Press, Glencoe, Illinois, 1964; E. Goffman, *Asylums,* Penguin, Harmondsworth, 1961; B. S. Georgopoulos and A. Matijko, 'The American General Hospital as A Complex Social System', *Health Services Research,* Spring 1967, pp.76-112. For observations about the difficulty of a patient group gaining even the rights laid down by government see M. Stacey *et al., Hospitals, Children and their Families,* Routledge and Kegan Paul, London, 1970.

44. Ann Cartwright, *Patients and their Doctors,* Routledge and Kegan Paul, London, 1967, p.216.

45. Winifred Raphael, *Patients and Their Hospitals,* King Edward's Hospital Fund for London, London, 1969.

46. R. Kohn and K. L. White (eds.), *Health Care: An International Study,* Oxford University Press, London, 1976.

47. Ann Cartwright, *Human Relations and Hospital Care,* Routledge and Kegan Paul, London, 1967.

48. E. L. Koos, *The Health of Regionville,* Hafner Publishing Co., New York, 1954.

49. Eliot Freidson, op. cit., 1961.

50. Julius Roth, *Timetables: Structuring the Passage of Time in Hospital and Other Careers,* Bobbs-Merrill, Indianapolis, 1963.

51. Fred Davis, *Passage Through Crisis: Polio Victims and Their Families,* Bobbs-Merrill, Indianapolis, 1962.

52. M. Bloor and G. Horobin, 'Conflict and Conflict Resolution in Doctor/Patient Interactions' in C. Cox and A. Meade (eds.), *A Sociology of Medical Practice,* Collier-Macmillan, London, 1975.

53. Lee and Gunawardena, this volume.

54. There is a great deal of anecdotal support for the contention that prescribed

régimes are ignored or modified. Two studies which provide more substantial evidence are: J. B. McKinlay, 'Social Networks and Utilization Behaviour', paper presented to the Second Social Science and Medicine Conference, 1970; C. R. B. Joyce, 'Patient Co-operation and the Sensitivity of Clinical Trials', *Journal of Chronic Diseases,* 15, 1962, pp.1025-36.

55. D. Robinson, op. cit., 1971.

56. The presentation of social life as a drama is a metaphor frequently employed by those sociologists who are particularly interested in explaining 'social action' and social processes. The work of Erving Goffman (e.g. *Asylums, Presentation of Self in Everyday Life, Stigma,* etc.) is a good example, so too is G. J. McCall and J. L. Simmons, *Identities and Interactions,* Free Press, New York, 1966.

57. G. Stimson and B. Webb, *Going to See the Doctor, The Consultation Process in General Practice,* Routledge and Kegan Paul, 1975, pp.26-7.

58. Since the Second World War there has been a spate of studies concerned with working-class deference: J. H. Goldthorpe, D Lockwood, F. Bechhofer and J. Platt, *The Affluent Worker in the Class Structure,* Cambridge University Press, Cambridge, 1969; W. G. Runciman, *Relative Deprivation and Social Justice,* Routledge and Kegan Paul, London, 1966; R. McKenzie and A. Silver, *Angels in Marble,* Heinemann, London, 1968; E. A Nordlinger, *The Working Class Tories,* McGibbon and Kee, London, 1967; and many others.

59. Howard Newby, 'The Deferential Dialectic', *Comparative Studies in History and Society,* 17, 2, April 1975.

60. Erving Goffman, 'The Nature of Deference and Demeanor', in his *Interaction Ritual,* Penguin University Books, Harmondsworth, 1972.

61. In order to avoid repetition of argument and material in Chris Ham's paper in this volume, no detailed discussion of the effectiveness of the health-related pressure groups is offered. None the less it is worth noting his point that the major pressure groups have adopted a more thrusting position. This is in part a reflection of the greater acceptability of the 'consumer ethic' and it is also a manifestation of the need felt by the voluntary organisations to return to the forefront of social policy. Having for a long time provided services supplementary to the NHS which have sometimes shored up bad policies and practices, they have turned to more fundamental questioning. So far these questions and the proposals which flow from them have fallen short of any real criticism of the structural position of health professionals. The Patients' Association and some of the CHCs have begun to take this line.

62. It is interesting that Royal Commissions were established in 1976 to look into both legal and medical practice. Both professions are acutely unhappy about their own representation on these enquiries. Editorials and features in the professional press have developed an hysterical and almost persecuted strain which reflects anxiety about the tenor of public debate about their role. The medical profession at the time of writing seems to feel itself under pressure of public criticism and governmental policies adverse to their interests. The editorial 'Priorities and Morale in the NHS', *BMJ,* 12 June 1976, is one symptom of this position. In his conclusion the editorial writer says: 'Surely the DHSS should be on the side of doctors and other health workers, and not seen as hostile to "them". Furthermore, the government must tell the public why NHS standards may fall. Otherwise doctors and other health workers, will take the brunt of patients' inevitable discontent...'

63. David Mechanic, 'Correlates of Frustration among British General Practitioners', *Journal of Health and Social Behaviour,* 11, 2, 1970, pp.87-104.

64. Eliot Freidson, op. cit., 1970.

65. C. M. Boyle, 'Differences between Patients' and Doctors' Interpretations of

some common Medical Terms', *BMJ*, 2, May 1970, and reprinted in C. Cox and A.Meade (eds.), *A Sociology of Medical Practice*, Collier-Macmillan, London, 1975.

66. Ann Cartwright and Maureen O'Brien, 'Social Class Variations in Health Care and the nature of General Practitioner Consultations', in M. Stacey (ed.), *The Sociology of the NHS*, Sociological Review Monograph 22, Keele, March 1976.

67. J. Tudor Hart, 'The Inverse Care Law', *The Lancet*, 27 February 1971, and reprinted in C. Cox and A.Meade, op. cit., 1975.

68. Mary Ann Elston, this volume.

69. Stuart Dimmock, this volume.

70. Davies Committee, *Report of the Committee on Hospital Complaints Procedure*, HMSO, London, 1973.

71. Jack Hallas, *CHCs in Action*, Nuffield Provincial Hospitals Trust, London, 1976. See also the less optimistic but rather early observation in R. Klein and J. Lewis, *The Politics of Consumer Representation, A Study of Community Health Councils*, Centre for Studies in Social Policy, London, 1976.

72. Observation of CHCs in action suggests that the more effective ones have already proved themselves capable of substantially affecting the allocation of resources and the conduct of medical, nursing and administrative practice. A few have uncovered malpractices, others have shifted money into psychiatry, geriatrics or the chronically ill. All are involved in planning procedures in some way.
    In the early months the more assertive CHCs came to public notice because of their attacks on the system. But most of their day-to-day work is concerned with improving effectiveness within the existing confines of policy and resources.

73. Malcolm L. Johnson, 'Whose Stranger Am I? Or, Patients Really are People' in K. A. Barnard and K. Lee (eds.), *NHS Reorganisation: Issues and Prospects*, University of Leeds/Frances Pinter, 1974; J. Hallas, *Mounting the Health Guard: A Handbook for Community Health Councils*, Nuffield Provincial Hospitals Trust, London, 1974.

74. Margaret Stacey, 'The Health Service Consumer: A Sociological Misconception' in M. Stacey (ed.) *The Sociology of the NHS*, Sociological Review, Monograph 22, Keele, 1976.

5 POWER, PATIENTS AND PLURALISM

Chris J. Ham

In both capitalist and non-capitalist countries the state has increasingly dominated the lives of individuals in the course of this century. Associated with this development, and in part a consequence of it, numerous groups have been formed to represent the interests of individuals to the state. Many political scientists now look on the group rather than the individual as the basic unit of political life, especially in Western industrialised societies where group formation is at its most advanced.[1]

In these societies, the pluralist theory of democracy has emerged as the dominant explanation of the way in which political power is distributed and structured. This theory holds that power is not concentrated in a single homogeneous class or élite, but rather is shared between a multiplicity of groups, including official or governmental groups. As argued by one of its principal exponents, Robert Dahl,[2] the theory states that although there are inequalities in the distribution of power, any group can make its voice heard effectively at some stage in the decision-making process. Dahl further contends that a group is heard effectively when 'one or more officials. . . expect to suffer in some significant way if they do not placate the group, its leaders, or its most vociferous members'.[3]

Pluralist theory is based on the twin premises that the sources of political power—money, time, status, information, expertise, charisma, and the like—are distributed non-cumulatively; and that no one of these sources dominates the others. Hence, no group is totally excluded from having a voice in decision-making as each group has some resources that enable it to exercise power. On the other hand, no group dominates decision-making, and while a group may get its preferences adopted in one issue area, it will not be able to do this in others. Consequently, in a pluralistic political system, power is fragmented and diffused.

This conclusion has been challenged by several writers, who take issue with the pluralists on a number of grounds. For instance, it is argued that the definition of power used is incomplete, and that the methodology adopted by the pluralists is inadequate. Again, the theory's descriptive validity has been questioned in view of the poor organisation of some sections of society, and the apparent inability of those sections to influence decision-making. An argument often heard is

that certain interests—the poor, ethnic groups, women and consumers
are the ones most frequently mentioned—have not been able to form
strong organisations to represent their demands to government, and that
their voices have not been heard effectively. One explanation of this is
that political resources are distributed cumulatively, not non-
cumulatively as pluralists maintain. Criticisms such as these have cast
doubts on the general applicability of the pluralist model.[4]

Ideas derived from pluralist theory have been applied in various
studies of the National Health Service.[5] The Service provides a fertile
testing ground for some of the claims and counter-claims identified
above because it comprises different and sometimes conflicting
interests: producer interests such as doctors, nurses, the para-medical
professions, ancillary workers and administrators; comsumer interests
in the form of patients, potential patients and patients' relatives; and
the politicians vested with formal authority for directing the Service and
with their own ideas about the way in which health care should be
delivered.

Elsewhere in this volume some of the problems currently facing producer groups and politicians are discussed.[6] In this paper attention is
focused on patients' groups in an attempt to examine both the pluralists' contention that any group can make itself heard effectively, and
the opposing view that interest groups like consumers exercise little or
no influence on decision-making because they lack political resources.

As an aid to understanding the position of organised patients today,
consumer representation through the Regional Hospital Boards (RHBs)
and Hospital Management Committees (HMCs) which administered the
largest part of the NHS between 1948 and 1974, will be considered first.
The experiences and prospects of Community Health Councils will then
be scrutinised in an examination of some of the issues of consumer
representation at local level. Finally, the spotlight will be directed at non-
statutory patients' pressure groups to discover how consumers' interests
are articulated nationally. The various strands of the paper will then be
drawn together in a consideration of the difficulties of establishing an
effective consumer voice in the NHS.

Regional Hospital Boards and Hospital Management Committees

When the NHS was established in 1948 one of the functions given to
RHBs and HMCs was the representation of consumer interests. To
quote from the Ministry of Health's Handbook for Members of Hospital Management Committees: 'the aim of the Management
Committee's work is to provide the best possible service to patients

within the means available,' and the same document described the HMC
as 'the body representing the consumer'.[7] Further, an early circular on
the subject urged Boards to consult 'organisations representing the
consumer interest' in appointing HMC members.[8] Clearly, then, the
Ministry saw Boards and Committees as representatives of patients.

Now there are at least three senses in which a group of people can be
said to be representatives.[9] Firstly, they can be freely elected, in which
case the selection procedure is the touchstone. As RHBs and HMCs
were appointed bodies, they were not representative in this sense.
Secondly, a group can be typical of the wider community, a microcosm
of the constituency from which its members are drawn. A survey conducted by the Fabian Society in 1964 looked into the composition of
a number of Boards and Committees, and found that their members
were quite untypical of the community.[10] The average age of RHB
members was 62; 81 per cent were male; and only one of the members
of the four Boards studied was an industrial worker. So on grounds of
age, sex and occupation the RHBs were unrepresentative because their
members were drawn from limited sections of the community. A similar
conclusion was reached with regard to Hospital Management Committees. The survey also revealed that over a quarter of the members of the
Boards belonged to the medical profession, and a key producer group in
the National Health Service was therefore in a good position to influence decision-making at that level.

The third sense in which RHBs and HMCs could be said to represent
patients would be if they were agents. In this case, 'irrespective of who
they are, how they are chosen, or how much discretion they are
allowed, their function is to look after the interests of the organisation,
group or person that they represent'.[11] Ambassadors are a good
example of this form of representation, and apparently this was also
how the Ministry envisaged Boards and Committees fulfilling their representative roles, since they were neither elected nor chosen because
they were typical of society. But how successful were they in doing
this?

Although it is not possible to give a definitive answer to this question,
there is evidence to suggest that they may have paid only lip service to
their duty to represent consumer interests. In view of their position in
the administrative structure of the Service, RHBs and HMCs were potentially a very important means of translating consumer opinions into
policy decisions. Yet in most cases they were seemingly unaware of
these opinions and made few efforts to find out what local communities
felt about the health services provided in their areas.

Nowhere was this more thoroughly documented than in the series of reports into conditions at mental hospitals—Ely, Farleigh, South Ockendon and Whittingham—and the criticisms contained therein of RHBs and HMCs.[12] To cite just one example, the Ely enquiry stated: 'the HMC responsible for Ely has lacked the necessary enthusiasm or experience or awareness of what can and should be achieved and has failed to adopt a sufficiently dynamic approach to its task.'[13] The result of this neglect was, as is now known, the ill-treatment of patients.

All of these reports attributed at least some of the blame to the 'system'. They spoke of confusion as to the respective functions of members and officers, the proliferation of committees and sub-committees, and the lack of training for HMC members. A complicating factor was undoubtedly the combination of management and representative duties in hospital authorities. Not only were they required to represent the consumer but also they were expected to manage the service, and in most cases the latter undoubtedly took precedence. Symptomatic of this greater concern with management was an influential report on the administrative practices of Scottish hospital boards published in 1966. The report dealt almost exclusively with the management functions of boards, making only passing references to their role as 'consumer councils'.[14]

It is interesting to note therefore that in the reorganised National Health Service which came into operation in April 1974, management and representation have been separated. The Regional Health Authorities (RHAs) and Area Health Authorities (AHAs) which replaced RHBs and HMCs have been given an explicitly managerial brief, and their members have been chosen mainly for their managerial abilities. Although the present government has modified this approach by proposing to enlarge these authorities to make room for additional representatives of local NHS staff and local authorities, the split between representation and management largely remains intact.[15] In the reorganised NHS, Community Health Councils (CHCs) have been given the remit of representing the patient and their experience and prospects will now be considered.

Community Health Councils

The sparse terms of reference specified for CHCs in the 1973 Act—'to represent the interests in the health service of the public in the district' —were later amplified by a DHSS circular which enumerated a number of specific matters which CHCs might tackle.[16] The items listed included investigation of catering facilities, waiting periods, visiting hours and the like; comment on, and criticism of, AHA plans; and helping patients with complaints and complaints procedure. In short, a major part of the job of a CHC is to act as a pressure group on behalf of health care consumers. And again, since the members of CHCs are neither directly elected nor chosen for their typicality, but instead are nominated and appointed by local authorities (one-half), regional health authorities (one-sixth), and voluntary organisations (one-third), they are only representative in the sense of being agents of the community.

There has, however, been much heart-searching among councils as to how they can ensure that they are truly representative. Several means of securing greater public involvement have been tried, with varying degrees of success.[17] Concern with this problem stems mainly from the fear that CHCs will not be taken seriously by Health Service managers unless they are seen to be responsive to and representative of the views of their communities. That this fear is well grounded is shown by a recent survey of the attitudes of chief administrators of health authorities, who doubted whether CHCs were representative.[18]

The same survey also revealed that chief administrators felt that CHCs 'tended to see themselves as part of management'. This tendency is at the root of the second problem which CHCs have had to tackle: what role they should adopt in their relationship with health authorities. One source has contended that if CHCs are the patients' watchdogs they are faced with the choice of becoming 'snivelling lapdogs or rabid curs'.[19] The assumption here is that if CHCs are not against the Health Service establishment then they must be for it. But experience has shown this to be a false dilemma, and many CHCs have taken a middle line in which they are neither subservient nor aggressively independent. This role has been termed that of 'a critical friend'.[20] A more accurate typology would therefore contain a spectrum of roles, ranging from conflictual through constructively critical to consensual.

A number of councils have uncompromisingly identified themselves with the communities they have been set up to represent, and have placed the emphasis on 'acting in the interests of ordinary people'[21] and challenging the power of professionals. Others, while not actively seeking conflict, have not held back from criticism when they have felt this has been deserved, and have carefully avoided becoming too closely associated with management. But the majority of CHCs have tended towards the consensual end of the role spectrum. They exhibit many of the attitudes formerly associated with HMCs, are deferential to officers, believe they have to earn the respect of those in authority, and espouse a philosophy which emphasises responsibility. Thus, the author of a review of the early experiences of CHCs in the north of England commented: 'If there is one generalization that is unfair to some, but, I think, justified by many, it is that on the whole councils have been far too polite and deferential.'[22]

It is not difficult to suggest reasons for this. In an organisation as complex as the NHS the expert is pre-eminent and the lay member at a disadvantage, and there is a strong temptation for CHCs to become consensual bodies. It is so much easier for councils to take on the job of a complaints' bureau-cum-hospital visiting committee rather than accept the challenge to become critical enquiring consumers' champions. Likewise, in the face of obstruction and delay by managers it is entirely understandable that CHCs may decide it is not worth the effort continuing to put up a struggle.

Judging by their annual reports, nearly all councils have experienced some unhelpful behaviour by managers: information has been withheld, consultation has occurred too late or not at all, and membership of health care planning teams, where sought, has been denied.[23] Again, the chief administrators' survey revealed that managers themselves have serious doubts about the part to be played by CHCs: the latter are seen as having power without responsibility and as being unwilling to do background work on problems referred to them. Indeed, those closest to CHCs, district administrators, 'were markedly more pessimistic than their Regional and Area colleagues about the Community Health Councils' effectiveness as consumer councils or in planning matters'.[24] While this is clearly not unbiased evidence, it does highlight the difficulties councils have faced in their search for a role separate from that of management.

Similar difficulties have confronted consumers' councils in the nationalised industries. There have been several studies of these councils, all of which have concluded that they have not been effective in representing consumer interests.[25] The main points made in these studies are that consumer councils are known by only a small proportion of the people they are intended to help; that they lack the information, technical expertise and research capability to critically examine proposals on which they are asked to comment; that they have 'no real power, but at most the right to know, to think, and to utter';[26] and that they tend to be subservient to the nationalised industry concerned, communicating producers' viewpoints to consumers instead of the reverse, and reacting to plans from above rather than formulating their own, alternative, policies.

Many of these points are relevant to CHCs. Firstly, despite strenuous efforts they are still not widely known, and nearly every annual report bemoans this state of affairs. If they are justifiably to claim to represent patients, and are to remain non-elected, CHCs will have to continue to search for ways of involving the public in their activities. Secondly, it is questionable whether councils have the resources to intervene effectively in the planning and decision-making processes. Many commentators have drawn attention to the importance of information for CHCs, yet equally crucial are other sources of power like money, time and staff. In this respect it is pertinent to note that the majority of CHCs operate on an annual budget of £15,000 or less; the time which members can give is limited by their other commitments as members of local authorities or voluntary organisations; and most councils have a staff of two—a Secretary and his or her assistant.

On the other hand, CHCs do have one important power in the form of their ability to withhold approval from plans to close hospitals or change their use. If an AHA cannot obtain the approval of a CHC to such plans, then they are referred to the Secretary of State for decision. Again, some CHC members are able to make use of key contacts in local, and national, political arenas and the mass media to bring pressure to bear on health authorities. But in general there is a gross inequality in the distribution of resources between CHCs and the health authorities they are required to monitor, and for this reason it is doubtful whether councils can become the effective 'counter-bureaucracy'[27] which some see as being needed to countervail the power of professionals in the NHS.

A more likely development is that CHCs will become co-opted into the main structure of the Service. In 1974 the government put forward the proposal that CHC members should be appointed to serve on AHAs, but this was dropped after consultation because it was felt that it would undermine the independence of councils from management. More recently, however, the Minister of State, Dr Owen, suggested that CHCs might undertake quasi-managerial tasks in the field of health education and health care planning teams. Specifically, Owen said that CHCs

could be very important in orienting people towards a philosophy that health is not just something that is provided for by the NHS, but that each individual has a responsibility for his own well-being. They could help to promote understanding that some of the great advances in medicine have come through preventive measures.[28]

There is little doubt that if CHCs were to perform tasks like these their independence would be brought further into question.

At the same time, though, the government has referred to the need 'to develop CHCs into a powerful forum where consumer views can influence the NHS and where local participation in the running of the NHS can become a reality',[29] and has taken a number of steps designed to achieve this. Councils have been given observer status and speaking rights at AHA meetings instead of overlapping membership as originally proposed, and district management team spokesmen attend CHC meetings to answer questions when invited. Further, a conference is to be held in November 1976 to decide whether to form a National Association of CHCs. There are other ways in which councils could be strengthened. If their budgets were increased to enable them to employ research staff this would make CHCs more independent of the formal management structure as far as information is concerned, and would permit the mass of data that is already available to be ordered and presented in a digestible form. Again, among the membership less reliance might be placed on local authority nominees who often appear to regard CHC work as secondary to their major interests. Such heavily committed members could be replaced by others with more time to give to the work of the CHC.

Yet, to summarise, it is difficult to be optimistic about the chances of CHCs effectively representing consumer interests in the light of the roles they have so far adopted, the limited resources available to them, the attitudes of health service managers and experience of consumers' councils in nationalised industries. One is therefore left to look further afield, and the rest of this paper is taken up with a discussion of some of the non-statutory pressure groups which represent patients.

National Pressure Groups

Outside the formal administrative structure of the NHS there are numerous autonomous groups which exist either to serve or represent the consumers of health care. They range from the Abortion Law Reform Association (ALRA) at one end of the alphabet to the Women's Royal Voluntary Service (WRVS) at the other, and it may be said that these two groups are also at opposite extremes in so far as methods and aims are concerned. ALRA is a pressure group which seeks to promote changes in the law relating to abortion, while the WRVS, as its name implies, is a service organisation which carries out voluntary work for deprived sections of the community.

Yet many patients' groups manage to combine pressure group and service functions, even if the combination is sometimes uneasy. Age Concern and MIND are both good examples of groups which attempt to influence government decision-making as well as provide a service, the former for old people, the latter for the mentally ill and handicapped. And the specialised interests represented by these organisations illustrate the point that most groups in the health field concern themselves with a certain section of patients, whether it be epileptics, autistic children, spastics, or sufferers of eczema or multiple sclerosis. One of the few exceptions to this is the Patients' Association, which tries to represent the interests of all patients.

These three groups—Age Concern, MIND, and the Patients' Association—are among the better-known patients' organisations, and each will be considered to assess how effectively it represents the interests it champions so that some of the strengths and limitations of patients' pressure groups can be identified.

Age Concern

Age Concern, whose official title is the National Old People's Welfare Council, was founded in 1940 by various organisations who were concerned with the hardships created for the elderly by wartime evacuation. As its historian, Nesta Roberts, notes,[30] in its first year the group took an interest in pensions, accommodation, the care of the chronic sick and infirm and medical treatment, and these remain its chief concerns thirty-six years later. From the outset the group sought to monitor and co-ordinate existing services, pioneer new developments, and influence government decision-making. To help it in these tasks it encouraged the formation of local Old People's Welfare Committees, and today there are over 1,000 of these Committees in England. Like Age Concern nationally, local organisations bring together people who work with the elderly, academics with a special interest in the problems of old people, and voluntary workers who want to help the aged. They provide services such as day centres, clubs and voluntary visiting, and also seek to inform the elderly about their rights to statutory services.

Age Concern's national organisation supports and stimulates local groups, and draws on their experience and knowledge in formulating its own policies. It also finances projects beyond the scope of local groups, like the formation of an Age Concern Housing Association. In addition, the national organisation acts as an information clearing house and has produced numerous specialist and research reports and information leaflets. All of these functions can broadly be described as part of the servicing role of Age Concern; but in turn they are the foundation of its pressure-group activities.

From its earliest days Age Concern has recognised and acted on the need to change government policy as well as the need to monitor and co-ordinate it. Thus, it was one of the organisations which submitted evidence to the Beveridge Committee, and was especially active in the post-war years in pointing out gaps in the health and social services legislation of the Attlee government and its successors. But in the last five years added emphasis has been given to what is euphemistically termed 'social advocacy', and the adoption of the name Age Concern in 1971, along with the appointment of David Hobman as Director and the gaining of independence from the National Council of Social Service, heralded a noticeable change in style and gave a new impetus to the organisation's pressure-group role. The result is that Age Concern is now established as *the* pressure group for the elderly.

The three main channels through which all pressure groups operate are government departments, Parliament and the mass media. The first of these is the most important in as much as government departments are the main centres of decision-making in the British political system. Age Concern has a number of informal contacts in the Department of Health and Social Security and other Ministries with responsibilities for old people, and it encourages civil servants to attend its meetings as observers. By advocating and initiating alternative policies, as well as responding to requests for advice and information, the group has built up a useful working relationship at this level.

In contrast, contacts with MPs are haphazard, although an attempt is currently being made to instil new life into the moribund All Party Pensioners Group. Never the less, Age Concern has achieved successes in Parliament, as when it supported MPs who rebelled against the earnings rule in 1975, and it is usually able to find a sympathetic Member to put down a question or speak in a debate should the need arise.

The group has increasingly supplemented its actions through these two channels by putting over the case for an improvement in the status of the elderly through television and radio programmes and newspapers. Arguably this is the most significant aspect of Age Concern's work, as only by changing society's attitudes towards the old will the group's more specific attempts to influence policy-making be effective. Age Concern recognises this, and in its recently published 'Manifesto on the place of the retired and elderly in modern society' stated: 'It is. . . urgently necessary to educate the public mind in its attitude towards the elderly in order to banish, once and for all, the widely-held image of the old as passive, poor and pitiful second-class citizens.'[31]

But the very fact that the elderly can still be seen as 'second-class citizens' shows that the change in attitudes which Age Concern has campaigned to bring about has yet to be realised, and the question inevitably arises: how well equipped is Age Concern to carry through this educative process and to influence decision-making? The major resources available to the group are expertise and knowledge derived from experience in service provision and academic research. These have established Age Concern as a credible organisation which is in contact with the grass roots and at the same time aware of the latest developments in the care of old people. It commands respect among those interested in this area of public policy and has a reputation for being knowledgeable and informed. This is reflected in the financial support given by the DHSS, which in 1974 contributed £55,000 out of Age Concern's total income of £273,050. With this income 47 full-time and 11 part-time staff were employed. The group's respectability is enhanced by the impressive list of people who have associated themselves with its work, and these include the Duchess of Kent as Patron and Lord Seebohm as President.

Hence, Age Concern possesses a number of power sources and these have enabled it to make its voice heard effectively at various times in the decision-making process. One result may have been that, of late, greater priority has been accorded to geriatric services in the NHS.[32] Yet this achievement and others have not been won easily or rapidly. The fundamental reason for this is that while the group can make demands based on reasoned and informed arguments, it can do little to protest if these demands are rejected. Unlike producer groups in the NHS, Age Concern has no sanctions to invoke if its preferences are dismissed or simply ignored. Contrary to what the pluralist model asserts, it cannot make officials suffer in its attempts to achieve its goals. This is a basic deficiency which limits Age Concern's power in the decision-making process, and its ability to get its preferences adopted is therefore tightly circumscribed.

MIND

MIND, which is also known as the National Association for Mental Health, was established in 1946 by the amalgamation of three voluntary mental welfare bodies. Today, it co-ordinates and supports the work of around 140 local associations and steering committees for mental health, and its membership of over 11,000 contains a strong professional element.

Traditionally, under Mary Appleby's twenty-two years' leadership, MIND concentrated on providing services, emphasising the pioneering and innovatory aspects of its work. It attempted to complement rather than duplicate statutory provision, and to this end initiated and continues to run projects like group homes, sheltered accommodation and workshops, residential establishments, social clubs and self-help groups. A further facet of MIND's servicing function is the educational, advisory and training activities it organises: information packs for teachers and youth leaders have been prepared; a public information service gives advice on all aspects of mental health; and courses and conferences are run for professionals and interested lay members.

As in the case of Age Concern, these functions are combined with what are best described as pressure-group activities. And, again like Age Concern, in recent years these activities have been given more prominence. Between 1971 and 1973 David Ennals, the present Secretary of State, ran the MIND campaign which coupled fund-raising with an attempt to secure greater interest in mental health, and a more sympathetic public attitude towards mental illness and handicap. At the end of the campaign the name MIND was permanently adopted, and Tony Smythe became Director. Since then the additional stress which Ennals' efforts placed on the pressure-group role has been accentuated, and under Smythe's direction MIND has more clearly become a visible campaigning organisation.

This is evidenced by the group's withdrawal from the management of a number of its community homes; by the establishment late in 1975 of a Legal and Welfare Rights Service; and by MIND having become less identified with the interests of professionals and more concerned with the needs of patients. The group's traditional desire to pioneer and not duplicate has been underscored, and, in association with a feeling that MIND should not be doing the government's job for it, has been used to justify less involvement in service provision. Further, the move away from professionals' interests towards patients' rights has been prompted by a sense that in the past MIND has been associated too closely with the psychiatrists, nurses and social workers who are so prominent among its membership, and has too readily assumed a universality of interests between producers and consumers of mental health care.

As recently as 1973 one commentator asked why MIND had not exposed the ill-treatment of patients in mental hospitals before the series of investigations beginning with Ely were conducted, and accused the organisation of 'complacency' in its attitude towards the revelations. He went on to suggest that mental health pressure groups should show 'more clamour and militancy' and not be afraid of 'alienating [their] more conservative supporters'.[33] Nowadays the opposite charge is more commonly heard: it is claimed that MIND has gone to the other extreme, no longer cares about professionals, and is too astringent in championing patients' rights. This is indicative of the changes which have been wrought in the last three years under Smythe's leadership. More than any other patients' organisation in the National Health Service, MIND is now established as a vociferous, campaigning group.

This can be seen in the range of its political activities. On the basis of many years' experience, MIND has built up a close relationship with the Department of Health and Social Security, and the extent to which it is an established element in the Department's consultative network is illustrated by the frequency with which the group's comments and advice are solicited. For instance, MIND was specifically asked for its views on the White Paper 'Better Services for the Mentally Ill', the Davies Committee's Report on Hospital Complaints Procedure, and the Butler Committee's Report on Abnormal Offenders. In addition, it often initiates and proposes suggestions for change, as in its authoritative and comprehensive review of the working of the 1959 Mental Health Act.[34]

In Parliament the group has been energetically rebuilding the All Party Parliamentary Mental Health Group, which currently claims a membership of 170 peers and MPs. This group provides MIND with invaluable access to the legislature, and its members can be relied on to lobby Ministers, speak in debates and table questions. Nor has MIND neglected the mass media, especially since the MIND campaign was launched in 1971. One of the main aims of the campaign was to alter public attitudes in favour of the mentally ill and handicapped, to create a public pressure for change, and this work continues today.

A further channel of pressure is the courts, and MIND's new concern with legal rights has been prompted by Smythe's background at the National Council for Civil Liberties and the appointment of Larry Gostin as Legal and Welfare Rights Officer. In this connection, MIND is piloting a series of test cases through the courts to discover exactly what mental patients' rights are in various fields including education and voting.

Like Age Concern, MIND's pressure-group activities at all levels are grounded in experience drawn from service provision and an awareness of current research, and there are other parallels between the two groups. MIND too has a member of the Royal Family—Princess Alexandra— as Patron, and a peer—Lord Butler—as president. MIND also receives a government grant, which in 1974 amounted to £87,500 out of an income of £390,000. In the same year the group employed a total staff of 70. Yet in contrast with Age Concern, the juxtaposition of pressure-group and service functions in MIND is uneasy, mainly because of the greater weight the latter has lately attached to its pressure-group role, and there are recurrent internal debates about the speed and direction in which MIND should be moving.

Never the less, there are persuasive arguments in favour of a new strategy such as the one MIND is developing because mental health, along with geriatrics, remains one of the 'Cinderella' sectors of the NHS. While successive Ministers have accepted the need to devote a larger proportion of the Health Service budget to mental health, spending at the point of delivery has not matched Ministerial aspirations and declarations. However, whether MIND will be able to change this situation is open to doubt for the same reason that applied in the case of Age Concern: although the group possesses power sources, and while it can claim some successes in influencing decision-making, its lack of sanctions if its demands are rejected is an inherent weakness.

A related problem is that the more of a protest movement MIND becomes (and in 1972 Ennals wrote: 'We were certainly not created as a protest movement but, without reducing our pioneering and service roles, we have become one'[35]) the greater will be the difficulties in satisfying the different constituencies to which it appeals. At one and the same time the group has to attempt to: retain and add to the support of its own members; attract the attention of the mass media to its statements and demands; mobilise other sympathetic groups like MPs, the general public, and psychiatrists; and persuade decision-makers to adopt its preferences. There are numerous points of conflict here. To obtain time on television and radio and space in newspapers, MIND has to use tactics and make controversial declarations which may not be approved of by its members. Again, the more militant and critical it is of government, the more precarious its position in the consultative process becomes. And even if decision-makers are moved to action, their responses to protest are just as likely to be symbolic as tangible.[36] Hence, greater concentration on a protest strategy may make MIND more widely known, but it may not make the group more effective.

The Patients' Association

The Patients' Association is the youngest of the three groups under discussion here, having been started in 1963 in a period which also saw the formation of a number of 'specific' patients' pressure groups, such as the National Association for the Welfare of Children in Hospital. There are several reasons why the early 1960s saw an increase in the number of patients' groups, but perhaps the most important was the feeling that the administrative machinery of the National Health Service had failed to make adequate provision for consumer representation, and that the bias towards management in RHBs and HMCs, remarked on earlier in this paper, needed to be reversed. As the Patients' Association founder said in 1963, 'there is no one to represent the patient',[37] and it was to fill this gap that the group was formed.

Paradoxically, although the Association has the widest interests of all patients' groups, it also has one of the smallest memberships, just over 1,000 at the last count. Since it depends mainly on members' subscriptions for its income, this restricts the scope of its work, though in 1975, at the personal instigation of the Minister of State, Dr David Owen, it received a government grant, amounting to £1,500, for the first time. In all respects, therefore, it is the poor relation of Age Concern and MIND: it has one paid member of staff; a tiny office in central London (MIND's headquarters are in Harley Street, while Age Concern has recently moved to new accommodation in Mitcham); and few other resources except for the determination and vigour of its unpaid Chairperson, Jean Robinson.

On a smaller scale, the Association parallels Age Concern and MIND in combining servicing and pressure-group functions. By publishing information leaflets, advising on complaints and complaints procedure, and, in some cases, taking up problems on behalf of patients, the group provides a service; by commenting on government reports, issuing press statements, and presenting its views through the mass media, it attempts to influence decision-making. There are certain similarities between the Association's work and that of Community Health Councils, and Robinson initially believed the Association's days were numbered when CHCs were formed. Yet they continue to operate alongside one another, and judging by the reported heavy volume of correspondence and requests for help the Association receives there is still a place and a need for it.

Like other patients' groups, the Association was quick to recognise the potential importance of CHCs, and Robinson is herself a member of the Oxford CHC. Having also served on a regional hospital board, she speaks from some experience in asserting that the calibre of CHCs' members is superior to that of the now defunct hospital authorities.[38] The Association publishes a newsletter for CHCs entitled 'Patient Voice', and, in common with other autonomous pressure groups, seeks to permeate CHCs in an almost Fabian fashion. (Age Concern has also taken an interest in CHCs, and as well as having at least one member on most councils, has prepared two information packs specifically for health councillors.)

The niche which the Patients' Association has carved out for itself in the field of consumer representation would seem to owe much to the assertive and confident manner in which Jean Robinson speaks on medical matters. The energetic way she tackles her job has meant that the Association is reasonably well known despite its comparative smallness. And the group can claim successes in following up individual complaints, as well as in more general areas: establishing the right of patients in teaching hospitals to be treated without being used for educational purposes, contributing to the pressure which led to the establishment of the Health Services Commissioner, and participating in the campaign against induced births.

But the Association's ability to further improve the status of the patient is constrained by its lack of power sources. A group of its size cannot make its voice heard effectively in the decision-making process with any regularity. Like other patients' pressure groups, the only way the Association can get its preferences adopted is by the use of reasoned arguments. If these fail to convince decision-makers, the group is unable to take further action. This is indicated by a report in one of the Association's newsletters of a visit to DHSS, which stated: 'The Ministers were friendly and reasonably frank, though they seemed unlikely to give on points where they have resisted us! It was useful to have the chance to put our arguments.'[39] Thus, even more so than Age Concern and MIND, the group lacks the political resources needed if it is to have anything more than a marginal and intermittent effect on decision-making.

Conclusion

The preceding discussion has attempted to show that since the inception of the NHS patients' interests have been represented by a number of different groups. What is perhaps most characteristic of these groups is the variety of their organisation and behaviour: some aim to represent specific client groups, while others encompass patients as a whole; some are part of the statutory machinery of the Service, while others are outside that machinery; and some try to influence decision-making in a visible, campaigning style, while others prefer quieter, consensual methods.

One point which was noted in the discussion of RHBs and HMCs was the presence of members of the medical profession on hospital authorities, and this has been continued on Health Authorities since reorganisation. This element of syndicalism is also in evidence at the national level. Brown, for example, has observed that the consultative machinery on the health and welfare side of the Department of Health and Social Security 'tends to be dominated by those who provide services rather than those for whom services are intended', and he comments, 'there is little scope for populism or for consumerism within the formal machinery'.[40]

This is very largely a function of the distribution of power within the NHS, a pragmatic recognition on the part of decision-makers of where the power lies. There have been several studies of pressure groups in the NHS, all of which have concluded that the groups representing doctors exercise considerable influence over decision-making.[41] Being a key producer interest in the Service, doctors have a sanction—the ability to withhold their services—to support their demands. Coupled with control over information, this places the profession in a strong bargaining position. Recently, other producer groups, most notably ancillary workers and nurses, have also become conscious of the power sources they possess, and have used these sources to press their interests and in a number of cases achieve their goals.

In comparison, the consumers of health care are poorly placed. It is true that the groups representing patients do have political resources, and to this extent the pluralists' thesis is supported. However, they lack the means to make themselves heard effectively in the sense that 'one or more officials. . . expect to suffer in some significant way if they do not placate the group, its leaders, or its most vociferous members'. Patients' groups can argue a case in a reasoned and informed manner, but they do not have the resources to increase the pressure if decision-makers are unwilling to accede to their demands. They can attempt to persuade but cannot make threats of any great significance, and because of this officials know that the preferences of patients' groups can most often be ignored without severe consequences following.

In seeking to explain this it is necessary to recall the point made earlier that nearly all patients' organisations are representative in that they are agents. Put another way, they are groups for patients not groups *of* patients, and this is underlined by their preference for the term social advocate rather than pressure group.

But there are major, perhaps insuperable, obstacles to creating what might be termed a patients' union, or to building a stronger coalition of existing groups. Margaret Stacey has recently reiterated these obstacles: the majority of patients are short-stay and therefore intermittent; the minority who are not are those least able to take action—the chronic sick and the mentally disordered; neither long- nor short-stay patients are in a condition to organise themselves; in any case, the dominant ideology in the health care system accords a controlling role to the doctor and a passive, acquiescent, unquestioning role to the patient; there is a knowledge, and often a class, gap between producers and consumers; and in a state service such as Britain's the patient lacks choice.[42]

The problems of organising consumers are not peculiar to the Health Service. For instance, governments of both political parties have, in evolving prices and incomes policies, negotiated with representatives of workers and employers but not consumers, and only recently have consumers gained a place on the National Economic Development Council, through the statutory National Consumer Council. Similarly, although there are signs of an emerging claimants' movement, and while council tenants have achieved some degree of organisation, in general the recipients of welfare state provision have not been noticeably effective in forming groups to represent their interests. As noted elsewhere in this volume, there may be signs that this is changing and that consumerism is developing as a potent force in a number of fields.[43] But historically at least consumers have been slow to recognise and collectively assert their rights.

What, then, are the prospects for more effective consumer representation in the Health Service? The answer to this rests on another question, which is: is there something which can be identified as *the* consumer interest? Stacey has noted 'the lack of patient consciousness, the lack of a feeling that patients have problems in common which they should combine to do something about', and she attributes this to the inculcation of a 'false consciousness' by the producers of care.[44] Apart from the intrinsic difficulties of falsifying or even testing the false consciousness thesis, this explanation overlooks the vital point that there may not be such a thing as a single patient consciousness (however latent). Rather, the heterogeneity of patients, and the development of autonomous patients' pressure groups to date, suggests the existence of a number of distinct patient consciousnesses and interests.

In these circumstances it is difficult to see a basis for a patients' organisation to represent the average consumer. Like the man on the Clapham omnibus, it may be that this person exists only in the imagination. If this is indeed true, then it is more realistic to look in the future to the consolidation of the position of Community Health Councils, the further development of groups representing the major separate patient interests, and the formation of a strong umbrella organisation on the trade union paradigm. A 'patients' TUC', containing representatives of groups like the Patients' Association, Age Concern, MIND and the National Association for the Welfare of Children in

Hospital, as well as CHC members, would undoubtedly strengthen the voice of consumers at the national level. In view of the inherent difficulties in organising patients as opposed to organising for patients, this seems to be the most likely way of achieving more effective consumer representation in the NHS.

Yet even if this were to happen, patients would still lack the sanctions which have been identified as a major source of the power of producer groups. A theme running through this paper has been that in pursuing their goals producer groups in the Health Service can make officials (and thereby, it should be added, patients) suffer, whereas consumer groups cannot. The observations of S. H. Beer are germane here. Writing of pressure groups in general, Beer has noted that 'the political power of the producer group rests on its ability to refuse to perform its function' and he has pointed to the fact that 'producer groups do have sanctions. . . which can cause, to put it mildly, "administrative difficulties", and which, by anticipation, endow the group with bargaining power in its relations with government.'[45] Consumer groups do not have this power, which another writer has termed 'socio-economic leverage',[46] and it is difficult to see how they can acquire it.

This is not to say that these groups exercise no influence over decision-making, for as has been shown they do possess other resources and have achieved some successes. But more fundamentally their effectiveness, both in terms of their ability to secure major changes and to consistently exert pressure, is limited by their own weaknesses and by the determination of other groups to press their interests. Further, the discussion of producer groups has pointed up the significance of the performance of productive functions as a power source, and has thrown into sharp relief the inequalities between producer and consumer groups in the NHS.

In the light of these comments, the pluralists' contention that any group can make itself heard effectively at some stage in the decision-making process should be treated circumspectly. The conclusion intimated by this analysis is that some power sources are far more important than others and that patients' groups, because they do not have sanctions, face considerable difficulties in attempting to influence decision-making. This accords with the prognosis of the pluralists' critics, and again raises the problem of how far the NHS can be made more responsive to the expressed demands of patients, a problem which assumes greater significance in the face of the increasing militancy of producer groups in the Service. It would be ingenuous to believe that there are any easy answers to this problem, but it is to be hoped that the need to keep the NHS responsive to the consumers it exists to serve will not be obscured or overwhelmed by the search for administrative rationality and management efficiency which dominated the reorganisation debate and which is still high on the agenda today.

Notes

1. A. F. Bentley, *The Process of Government*, Harvard University Press, Cambridge, 1967, originally published in 1908, is regarded as a seminal work by students of group politics.
2. Dahl has developed this theory in a number of works, but see especially: *A Preface to Democratic Theory*, University of Chicago, Chicago, 1956; *Who Governs?*, Yale University Press, New Haven, 1961; *Pluralist Democracy in the United States*, Rand McNally, Chicago, 1967.
3. Ibid., 1956, p.145.
4. For criticisms of pluralist theory see: P. Bachrach and M. S. Barratz, *Power and Poverty*, Oxford University Press, New York, 1970; S. Lukes, *Power: A Radical View*, Macmillan, London, 1974; R. Miliband, *The State in Capitalist Society*, Quartet, London, 1973; K. Newton, 'A Critique of the Pluralist Model', *Acta Sociologica*, Vol. 12, 1969, pp.209-32; E. E. Schattschneider, *The Semi-Sovereign People*, Holt, Rinehart and Wilson, New York, 1960.
5. See, *inter alia*, H. Eckstein, *Pressure Group Politics*, Allen and Unwin, London, 1960; R. Klein, 'Policy Making in the National Health Service', *Political Studies*, Vol. 22, 1974, pp.1-14; R. Klein, 'Policy Problems and Policy Perceptions in the National Health Service', *Policy and Politics*, Vol. 2, 1974, pp.219-36.
6. S. Dimmock, 'Participation or Control? The Workers' Involvement in Management'; M. A. Elston, 'Medical Autonomy: Challenge and Response'; J. C. Sunderland, 'Health Administrators and the Jaundice of Reorganisation', all in this volume.
7. *Handbook for Members of Hospital Management Committees*, HMSO, 1967, p.11.
8. RHB (49) 143.
9. A. H. Birch, *Representative and Responsible Government*, Allen and Unwin, London, 1964, pp.13-17.
10. M. Stewart, *Unpaid Public Service*, Fabian Society, London, 1964.
11. A. H. Birch, op. cit., p.14.
12. *Report of the Committee of Inquiry into Allegations of Ill-Treatment of Patients and other Irregularities at the Ely Hospital, Cardiff*, HMSO, London, 1969, Cmnd. 3975; *Report of the Farleigh Hospital Committee of Inquiry*, HMSO, London, 1971, Cmnd. 4557; *Report of the Committee of Inquiry into South Ockendon Hospital*, HMSO, London, 1974, HC 24; *Report of the Committee of Inquiry into Whittingham Hospital*, HMSO, London, 1972, Cmnd. 4861.
13. *Ely Report*, p.110.
14. *Administrative Practice of Hospital Boards in Scotland*, Report by a Committee of the Scottish Health Services Council, HMSO, Edinburgh, 1966, The Farquharson-Lang Report, paras.35-45.
15. *Democracy in the NHS*, HMSO, London, 1974, contained the Labour government's proposals for changes in the membership of health authorities.
16. HRC (74) 4.
17. The concern which CHCs feel about the need to be representative is illustrated by the following comment, taken from the first report of the Cardiff CHC,

but typical of the sort of remark which can be found in nearly every annual report: 'Whilst CHCs are required to represent the interests of residents of the areas in health services provided, there can be no doubt that this of itself presents very considerable problems.' The methods which have been used to attract public interest include leafleting, talking to voluntary organisations, seeking press and local radio coverage, holding open meetings, acquiring high street premises and taking stands at exhibitions. The Burnley, Pendle and Rossendale CHC has been more successful than most in having an average attendance of 20 people at its public meetings. W. Ashworth and G. Mitchell, 'The CHC and its public', *The Hospital and Health Services Review*, June 1976.

18. *A Review of the Reorganised NHS*, Working Party of the Association of Chief Administrators of Health Authorities, December 1975, p.30.
19. *Patient Power, The First Year*, Wandsworth and East Merton CHC, p.1.
20. M. L. Johnson, 'Whose Stranger Am I? Or Patients Really Are People', pp. 80-92, in K. Barnard and K. Lee (eds.), *NHS Reorganisation: Issues and Prospects*, Nuffield Centre for Health Services Studies, University of Leeds, 1974.
21. See note 19.
22. J. Hallas, *CHCs in Action*, Nuffield Provincial Hospitals Trust, London, 1976, p.59.
23. See, for example, Sunderland CHC, Annual Report 1974/5; North Derbyshire CHC, Annual Report 1974/5; and City and Hackney CHC, Annual Report 1974/5.
24. Op. cit.
25. G. Mills and M. Howe, 'Consumer Representation and the Withdrawal of Railway Services', *Public Administration*, Vol. 38, 1960, pp.253-62; *Consumer Consultative Machinery in the Nationalised Industries: Report by the Consumer Council*, HMSO, London, 1968; *Relations with the Public: Second Report from the Select Committee on Nationalised Industries*, HMSO, London, 1971; *Consumers and the Nationalised Industries: Report by the National Consumer Council*, HMSO, London, 1976.
26. National Consumer Council, ibid., p.73.
27. R. Klein, 'Health Services: The Case for a Counter-Bureaucracy', pp.9-15, in S. Hatch (ed.), *Towards Participation in Local Services*, Fabian Tract, 419, 1973. Klein also draws a comparison with consumers' councils in national-ised industries and makes the point: 'As the experience of the nationalised industries has shown, there is little point in setting up consultative committees and all the other paraphernalia of participation if they then lack the independent resources to conduct a dialogue on equal terms. Similarly, it is difficult to be optimistic about the role of the proposed community health councils if they were to lack the means of measuring the performance of the services in their area against some benchmarks (however crude) of what was desirable from the point of view of the consumer and the best practices elsewhere.' (p.15)
28. *The Times*, 9 February 1976.
29. *Democracy in the NHS*, op. cit., p.17.
30. N. Roberts, *Our Future Selves*, Allen and Unwin, London, 1970.
31. *Manifesto*, Age Concern England, London, 1975, p.3.
32. *Priorities for Health and Personal Social Services in England*, HMSO, London, 1976.
33. B. Nightingale, *Charities*, Allen Lane, London, 1973, pp.207-8.
34. L. Gostin, *A Human Condition: The Mental Health Act 1959 to 1975*, MIND, 1975.
35. *MIND and Mental Health Magazine*, Summer 1972, p.29.

36. M. Lipsky, 'Protest as a Political Resource', *American Political Science Review*, Vol. 62, 1968, pp.1144-58, provides an interesting analysis of the mechanics of protest as a form of group behaviour, and concludes that it cannot be used with a high probability of success to extract tangible concessions from decision-makers. Lipsky suggests that instead decision-makers will make symbolic and other responses to protest, and his analysis is borne out by governmental decision-making in the mental health field. The White Paper, *Better Services for the Mentally Ill*, for instance, was presented as 'a long-term strategic document' which contained 'a statement of objectives against which shorter term decisions can be made' (HMSO, London, 1975, Cmnd. 6233). In no sense was it a programme to be achieved within a fixed term by the commitment of extra resources.

37. Quoted in B. Jerman, *Do something: A guide to self-help organisations*, Garnstone Press, London, 1971, p.95.

38. As quoted in *The Times*, 11 February 1976.

39. Newsletter 45, June 1975, p.1.

40. R. G. S. Brown, *The Management of Welfare*, Fontana, London, 1975, pp.193, 275.

41. See, *inter alia*, H. Eckstein, op. cit.; T. Marmor and D. Thomas, 'Doctors, Politics and Pay Disputes', *British Journal of Political Science*, Vol. 2, 1972, pp.421-42; N. Parry and J. Parry, *The Rise of the Medical Profession*, Croom Helm, London, 1976.

42. M. Stacey, *The Status of the Patient in the Health Service*, a paper given at the British Sociological Association's medical sociology group's conference on CHCs, at York, March 1976.

43. M. L. Johnson, 'Patients: Receivers or Participants?', in this volume.

44. Op. cit.

45. S. H. Beer, *Modern British Politics*, Faber, London, 2nd ed., 1969, pp.320, 331.

46. S. E. Finer, 'The Political Power of Organised Labour', *Government and Opposition*, Vol. 8, 1973, pp.391-406.

6 PARTICIPATION OR CONTROL? THE WORKERS' INVOLVEMENT IN MANAGEMENT

Stuart J. Dimmock

It can be suggested that the absence of overt forms of industrial conflict amongst hospital staff between 1948 and 1973 fostered the belief that the Health Service's labour relations were qualitatively different from those of industry: that the Service enjoyed a measure of insularity from the industrial relations issues which troubled other sectors of public and private industry. The series of industrial actions over pay that have occurred in the hospital sector since the ancillary workers' national wage dispute of 1973 indicate that the pattern of industrial relations has undergone a change. This paper is concerned to advance the following propositions. First, to suggest that the change in industrial relations represents an increasing awareness amongst Health Service staff, and in particular amongst ancillary workers, of their ability to exercise control over areas of decision-making that were the traditional reserve of hospital management. Second, to suggest that the proposals for increased participation that have emanated from the Department of Health and Social Security (DHSS) since the 1974 National Health Service Reorganisation may serve, unwittingly, to accelerate the exercise of staff control rather than to halt it. These proposals suggest that the DHSS may be clinging to the erroneous belief that the form and substance of Health Service industrial relations is different from industry; moreover, their implicit objective appears to be the containment of increased staff participation. It therefore seems that the DHSS may have failed to appreciate the lessons of industry or the nature of worker participation and its implications for collective employee behaviour in circumstances of developing workplace organisation. Thus, the third and predominant aim of this paper is to explore the Service's fundamental attitude towards increased participation and to suggest possible developments which may follow from its introduction.

The discussion which follows is divided into four major sections. Section One is concerned with the definitional problem of participation. The term 'worker participation' has been variously described as, for example: 'collective bargaining', 'joint consultation', and 'industrial democracy'. In consequence, this section advances a definition of worker participation to enable a clearer examination of its operation in the Health Service. The proposals for participation do not constitute an entirely novel departure from previous industrial relations policies in the Health Service for two vehicles for worker participation—collective bargaining and joint consultation—have been operated in the Service since its inception in 1948. Thus, the second section is an examination of some of the features of collective bargaining and joint consultation arrangements in an attempt to determine the extent to which they have enabled genuine participation in management decision-making. Since it has been suggested that the 1973 national dispute of hospital ancillary workers marked a turning point in Health Service industrial relations, the third section discusses the underlying features of the dispute and their significance for management decision-making. The final section explores the Service's proposals for increased participation against the definition of participation; the experiences of the Health Service and industry; and the development of workplace organisation amongst hospital ancillary workers.

Worker Participation

The hospital sector which dominates the National Health Service is a labour-intensive undertaking. For with some 26,000 doctors, 330,000 nurses and midwives, 40,000 professional and technical staff, 60,000 clerical and administrative staff and 204,000 ancillary staff, labour costs consume approximately 70 per cent of total expenditure.[1] The layperson may still believe that health care is provided by doctors and nurses with the assistance of a small number of supporting staff. In reality, however, the provision of direct patient care is supported by a complex infra-structure made up of numerous occupational sub-groups many of whom possess highly specialised skills and knowledge. Moreover, many of these sub-groups have little direct contact with the patient and may often work in factory-like conditions. With a labour force of this scale and variety, it would appear axiomatic that the whole field of industrial relations would be of crucial concern to the Ministry of Health and its successor, the DHSS. In practice, however, the subject has received scant attention over the past twenty or so years either from within the Service or without.

Following NHS reorganisation in 1974, it has been proposed that there should be greater participation in management decision-making by the work-force. Firstly, in addition to the representatives of medical and nursing staff appointed to each Regional and Area health authority, it has been proposed that two extra members should be included, by election, from the remainder of the employees. Secondly, that there should be introduced, by agreement, a revitalised system of joint consultation with committees in organisational units of an appropriate size, e.g. Areas, Districts, and large hospitals. Lastly, it is proposed that health authorities adopt the notion of 'Participative Management', to increase job satisfaction and improve efficiency through the establishment of working groups to examine problems and difficulties that affect the provision of patient care. As previously stated, the term 'worker participation' does not readily lend itself to a precise definition and the text that follows explores the term in order to clarify the concepts involved.

In a society which has experienced the displacement of the owner-manager by complex industrial organisations, it has become increasingly difficult to apply the label 'worker'. It has been suggested that managers are those who are accountable for the work of their subordinates while 'workers' are accountable only for their own work. However, these are necessarily extreme definitions as only those at the very top or the very bottom of an organisational hierarchy could be thus described; the vast majority in between are hence partly managers and partly workers. The increasing size and complexity of many hospitals represents a similar development to that of industry. Traditionally, the size of hospitals and the relatively narrow range of occupational skills tended towards the adoption of a management style not unlike that of small family firms. The emergence of the concept of the District General Hospital and the growth in the absolute number of staff and the development of new skills amongst occupational groups marked a shift towards large and complex hospitals and a lengthening of the lines of formal authority. The creation of successive levels of managerial authority has led inevitably to a situation in which the majority of the service's staff, including the doctors, are partly managers and partly workers. Although it is accepted that increased participation will affect all occupational groups and different levels of management, the term 'worker' will be used in this essay to refer to those members of the hospitals' staff who primarily are accountable for only their own work, i.e. the ancillary workers.

The second problem of definition in the term 'worker participation' relates to the word 'participation'. Literature on the subject suggests that a definition should concentrate on at least three central issues; the nature of participation; the ability of workers to participate; and the form of participation. When describing the nature of participation, writers have used such terms as 'influence' [2] or 'taking part'. [3] In contrast, Tannenbaum uses 'control' and defines it as 'any process through which a person or group of persons determines (i.e. intentionally effects) what a person or group of persons will do'.[4] For example, if management informed its workers of its forward plans, they could claim that the work-force was taking part in the running of the organisation. However, the workers would not be genuinely participating in the sense of effecting the future actions of management, rather that management would be determining the actions of the work-force. Participation in the Health Service, therefore, will be examined in relation to the degree of control it allows the workers to affect management decision-making.

A second and closely related issue is the ability of the work-force to participate, that is to exercise the degree of control allotted to them in the participation process or to exceed it. For example, if workers are provided with information by management as an exercise in 'good communications', it can offer the work-force a potential for genuine participation: they may subsequently decide, albeit contrary to management intentions, to use the information as a basis for affecting the future actions of management. In their discussion of the pluralist nature of American politics, Bachrach and Baratz make the following point: 'to the extent that a person or group—consciously or unconsciously—creates or reinforces barriers to the public airing of policy conflicts, that person or group has power.'[5] This view of the exercise of power in political situations is equally relevant to a discussion of worker participation, for it tends to reflect the actions and attitudes of management towards the sharing of its decision-making powers and it emphasises the role of 'power' in worker participation.

The notion of power is fundamental to the concept of participation as it determines its nature, i.e. the degree of control that each side can exercise over the actions of the other. The work-force may only exercise control when it is aware both of the power context in which participation takes place and of its power to exercise control over management actions. In this context, then, power may be linked with coercion, namely the securing of compliance through the threat of sanctions.

This can be illustrated in circumstances where workers seek to alter an organisation's forward plans in opposition to management. At this stage, the threat of sanctions may play a major role in determining the eventual outcome in that the actions of both parties will tend to be guided by the assumptions each side makes about the balance of power between them. The critical factor in this situation, however, will not be

the actual balance of power between the parties but rather their perceptions of that balance. Thus, should workers attempt to exercise control
through the threat of, or the application of, sanctions subsequent
events may prove that they underestimated the power of management
resistance. Alternatively, management may overestimate the power of
the work-force and decide to treat with its employees. Therefore a more
precise concept of the role of power in worker participation would be
its *perceived capacity* to enable the exercise of control.

A third issue relates to the form of participation. A useful distinction
suggested by Lammers is between 'direct' and 'indirect' forms of participation.[6] An 'indirect' form implies a process in which subordinate
participants speak on behalf of their constituents with senior managers
about the organisation's general policy. The procedures are formalised
and outside agencies often do influence to some extent what goes on.
'Direct' participation, however, customarily entails that subordinate participants speak for themselves about work or the matters related to it; in
general, formalised procedures and external influences are normally
absent. In so far as both direct and indirect forms of participation (as
defined by Lammers) are at opposite ends of a contimuum, normally
both will involve an element of bargaining and a codification of rules to
a greater or lesser degree. Further, representatives or outside agencies
may intervene in direct participation, while subordinates may take a
spontaneous decision to speak directly to top management.

In summary, then, genuine as opposed to token participation in
either a direct or an indirect form enables the workers to exercise a
degree of control over the actions of management. In consequence, the
concept of power is an inherent feature of participation: for in circumstances where management are reluctant to accord the work-force a
degree of control over decision-making, the workers may only achieve
participation through the threat or the application of sanctions. With
this exposition of the concept of worker participation in mind, the
National Health Service's previous experiences can be examined in an
attempt to determine the degree of control that it afforded to the work-
force.

Participation in the National Health Service, 1948 to 1973

The forms which participation in the Health Service have taken since
1948 have been in terms of collective bargaining and joint consultation
arrangements, both of which are indirect forms of participation. While
joint consultation has been the object of enquiry, there has been little
research to date on Health Service collective bargaining. However, one

measure of its effectiveness as a vehicle for participation is the extent
to which the staff side representatives have been able to control the process of negotiations. As a crude indicator this can perhaps be judged by
the incidence of independent arbitration as detailed below.

Collective Bargaining

The essence of the Service's approach to collective bargaining is a strong
belief in the efficacy of industry-wide joint agreements for the regulation
of pay and conditions of employment — the 'formal system' characterised
in the report of the Royal Commission on Trade Unions and Employers'
Associations, 1968.[7] As such, the underlying philosophy of the Service's
system of Whitley Councils reflects the views on industrial relations of
the Whitley Committee,[8] established in 1916, from which the Service's
collective bargaining arrangements took their name. The considered
opinion of the Whitley Committee was that a permanent improvement
in the relations between employers and employed could best be secured
by adequate organisation on both sides, and the establishment of industry-
wide agreements in which pay, hours of work and other conditions of
employment appropriate to regulation could be settled.

The suggestion that this could be achieved by the creation of Joint
Industrial Councils met with a positive response from both public and
private sectors of employment. While the number of Councils in industry declined after 1921, they continued to operate in areas of
government employment. The Civil Service National Whitley Council
set up in 1919 subsequently served as a model for negotiating arrangements that were later established in other government departments. One
such set of arrangements was the Health Service's system of Whitley
Councils[9] which in 1948 was forged from the patchwork of existing
arrangements. There was, however, at least one vital difference from the
Civil Service model. In Health Service Whitleyism, the Treasury was not
represented on the management side. Although the government is not
the formal employer of the Service's staff, it has, nevertheless, to provide the money to pay for wage increases and improvements in
conditions. The role played by the Treasury in collective bargaining is
therefore of significant importance and it must be assumed that it
plays a primary part in advising the amount which management sides
may offer in negotiations. Although its advice does not have to be
accepted, the doctrine of Cabinet solidarity and the powerful position
of the Chancellor suggests that Treasury advice is rarely seriously
challenged.[10]

Health Service Whitleyism has long been subject to criticism from

both the management and the staff. Management criticism has centred
on the remoteness of the central machinery from the actual workplace
and the slowness of its communications with the constituent employing
authorities. Trade unions, on the other hand, have frequently voiced
their frustration over their inability to talk directly with the Service's
paymaster, and the slowness of negotiations due to the absence of the
Treasury and the need for the departmental representatives to consult
it at successive stages in the negotiations. However, it should not be concluded that the positions of the management sides are solely determined
by the Treasury. There are other considerations, not least of which are
the implications of Health Service joint agreements for some local
authority employees, whose pay and conditions are often compared for
collective bargaining purposes. However, if there is a conscious policy on
Health Service pay it must ultimately be formulated by the Treasury, or
by the DHSS in conjunction with Treasury officials.

The inability of the staff sides to conclude successful pay claims in
Whitley Councils dominated by the absent Treasury has been noted by
Clegg and Chester, who remarked that although it was possible for the
staffs' representatives to persuade management to revise their offers, in
the end decisions have been offers of the management side accepted
by the staff, or the awards of arbitrators.

The frequent recourse to arbitration is an interesting and recurrent
feature of collective bargaining in the Health Service. There were 53
'major' settlements in the service from 1948 to 1955 and of these, 26
were the result of arbitration.[11] Moreover, the incidence of arbitration
continued throughout the late 1950s and early 1960s and by 1963 the
total number of referrals stood at 135.[12] Although the use of arbitration has declined since that period due to successive wage legislation,
important pay settlements have continued to be awarded outside the
Whitley framework.[13] The most likely explanation for this consistent
use of independent arbitration is that it provided a useful expedient
for successive governments whose economic policies require that they
should not be seen to be granting, too freely or readily, pay concessions
to their own employees. On the staff side, the variety of occupational
groups and the emphasis on professionalism militated against the formulation of a common policy for the total labour force, and, moreover,
the absence of strong collective organisation in hospitals served to
undermine the credibility of any threats by the staffs' national representatives to impose sanctions in support of pay claims. Therefore Health
Service employees in general, in that they perceived they were unable to
exercise effective control through the threat or the application of

sanctions, resorted to outside arbitration.

In contrast, one occupational group, the doctors, were in a position to exert control within the collective bargaining process. Klein has pointed to the major role played by the doctors, in spite of their small numbers, in Health Service policy-making.[14] The source of their power is based on their position within the policy-making structure which, in turn, is derived from the profession's control of medical expertise.[15] Unlike other occupational groups, the doctors were aware of their powerful position within the Service. Moreover, they were prepared to use that power to develop a separate channel for the determination of pay and conditions and, with the use of active lobbying, succeeded in getting their views on remuneration considered.[16]

Notwithstanding the collective bargaining behaviour of doctors and the frequency of arbitration for other occupational groups, Health Service Whitleyism, on the whole, has enabled government to exercise a large measure of control over the actual earnings of the Service's employees. It has, therefore, achieved one of the essential, if unwritten, objectives of Whitleyism—the containment of salary and wage costs in a labour-intensive industry. The conclusions of the Prices and Incomes Board Report No. 29,[17] that the Health Service contained large concentrations of low-paid manual workers, is sufficient demonstration of the extent to which Whitleyism had achieved this implicit objective, particularly in regard to hospital ancillary workers.

Joint Consultation

The other form of indirect participation, joint consultation, was introduced in 1950, though it too can be said to have a philosophy originally expounded by the Whitley Committee, who wrote in 1917, 'there are also many questions closely affecting in no small degree efficiency of working, which are peculiar to the individual workshop and factory.' They proposed works committees 'to establish and maintain a system of co-operation in all these workshop matters', but not to deal with 'questions such as rates of wages and hours of work'.[18] The Joint Consultative Committees that the Health Service's General Whitley Council recommended should be established in 'all hospitals within the National Health Service' were intended 'to promote the closest co-operation and provide a recognised means of consultation' between Hospital Management Committees (or their equivalent) and their senior officers, and the staff.[19] Further, two of the most common arguments for the introduction of participation, i.e. as a means of promoting job satisfaction and increased efficiency,[20] are specifically mentioned in the

General Council's constitution for joint consultation:

> to give the staffs a wider interest in and a greater responsibility for
> the conditions under which their work is performed; to give the
> maximum assistance in promoting the welfare of the patients and
> efficient administration in the hospitals.[21]

The extent to which the staff could exercise control in joint consultation is also spelt out in some detail; consultative committees could only
make recommendations which did not conflict with or override any
decisions of the industry-wide agreements. The constitution was equally
concerned to protect the prerogatives of hospital management: 'hospital authorities are free to withhold ratification if they think fit and so
prevent a recommendation of the Consultative Committee from
becoming operative.'[22]

The nature and form of the Service's consultative arrangements can
be compared with the main features of joint consultation in Britain.
Writers have pointed to the paradoxical attitude of management
towards joint consultation, which recognises a conflict of interest over
wages and hours of work and is prepared to accept that they be subject
to agreement, but which does not accept joint determination on other
matters that are deemed to be of common interest (e.g. the introduction
of new equipment or working arrangements), and maintains that they
are the sole prerogative of management. As McCarthy has stated: 'we
reach a position in which it is suggested that agreements are only possible when the two sides are basically opposed; when they are really
united there cannot be any question of agreement.'[23] The fate of joint
consultation in much of British industry has been to suffer a general
decline in proportion to the growth of workplace bargaining. In short,
industrial workers who have perceived that they have an ability to control management decision-making have pursued informal and *ad hoc*
forms of direct and indirect participation and have escaped the constric-
tions of joint consultation largely by ignoring it.

Joint consultation in the Health Service, however, was not overtaken
by workplace bargaining as it was already largely moribund within a
few years of its introduction. Even the conditions of its birth were less
than auspicious. In a series of negotiations between 1948 and 1950, the
management side of the General Council insisted that the membership
of committees should not be restricted to elected representatives of
nationally recognised negotiating bodies. Following an agreement which
accepted the staff side's view of this principle of exclusivity,

management urged, against the staff's wishes, that the constitution should be issued with a recommendation: 'That the Minister should advise the adoption of the constitution.'[24] Although the final outcome was again in favour of the staff, knowledge of these clashes had filtered down to hospitals, and this tended to reinforce the attitude of some hospital managements who believed that joint consultation had been foisted upon them by the centre without due consideration of their views.

Miles and Smith, in their history of joint consultation in the Health Service, have suggested that its early failure was due to a number of factors: a general lack of commitment among hospital managements; complete absence of any training for representatives in the concept and skills necessary for consultation to become effective; the reluctance of the General Council to respond to enquiries for further guidance from enthusiastic hospital authorities; and the refusal by the doctors to participate on the consultative committees. The doctors' rejection of joint consultation is perhaps the critical factor in its failure, and their action reflected the attitudes and behaviour of organised industrial workers towards this form of participation. As the one occupational group who was aware of its power, the doctors had obtained separate representation at hospital level in the shape of a Medical Advisory Committee (MAC) to the Hospital Management Committee. Moreover, the position of these MACs was further reinforced by the inclusion of medical representatives on Hospital Management Committees. Equipped therefore with an adequate forum for participation, it was unlikely that they would wish for involvement in a form of consultation which, by its nature, was superfluous to their needs.

The remainder of the staff, ill-organised and unconscious of their power, were thereby denied the support of the doctors and had to accept the operation of joint consultation on hospital managements' terms. The record suggests that these terms were based on a preference not to have participation. Thus, following the 1950 recommendation to some 400 hospital committees and boards to establish consultative committees, Miles and Smith's survey of 197 hospitals, published in 1969, revealed that 92 had admitted that no attempt had been made to start consultation, 29 had declined a statement or were covered by a subgroup organisation in which consultation was not easy, and 76 had indeed set up these committees. Of these 76, only 19 had survived through to 1963. Ironically, in 1952 in what appears to be the last official reference to joint consultation, the Ministry of Health commented:

The scheme was launched in the Summer of 1950 and since then joint consultative committees have been started in hospitals throughout the country. Over a considerable part of the hospital service the institution of these committees represented a new departure in the relationship between management and staff and time must be allowed before their effectiveness can be assessed. In the hospital where the common aim of management and staff, the recovery and well-being of the patients, is apparent to all, joint consultative committees start with every advantage and they should make an effective contribution towards the achievement of an harmonious and efficient service.[25]

The fact that the number of consultative committees were already in decline at the time of the Ministry's statement gives substance to management's criticisms about the remoteness of Whitleyism. More important, however, it highlights the differences that can occur between theory and practice, for it underlines a fundamental conflict in the Service's industrial relations policy-making. The sheer size and scope of the Health Service in terms of geography, organisation and labour (costs) have dictated that wages and general industrial relations policies be controlled by the Minister with Treasury involvement. However, the factors that have prompted the adoption of a system of centralised control often militate against its effective operation. They may require, moreover, a flexibility of approach that is beyond the capacity of centralised control. The 1952 Report's comments on joint consultation are an example of this fundamental conflict between the desire to provide centralised control whilst still retaining sufficient flexibility to respond to individual circumstances.

In summary, the absence of sustained efforts by the majority of the staff to exert a measure of control within either the collective bargaining or joint consultative arrangements led governments and the Service's management to regard industrial relations as a low-key activity. The extended period of industrial peace from 1948 to 1973 fostered and reinforced two basic beliefs about labour relations in the Health Service. One, that its objectives, the care of the sick, served to unify the workforce and to discourage industrial action which could be seen as being detrimental to the patient. Two, that the Whitley system had the ability to regulate effectively almost all aspects of the employment relationship. These two beliefs taken together could, it was felt, explain the absence of conflict and the seeming difference in the substance and form of Health Service industrial relations from that of industry.

Moreover, the supposed efficacy of Whitleyism as an instrument of management control led to a complacent assumption among many hospital managements that industrial relations *per se* were not a matter for local concern. For example, a survey of large hospitals in the London area conducted in 1971 showed that many senior managers believed that industrial relations were the responsibility of Whitleyism and the central authority.[26] The unprecedented upsurge of industrial action across a range of occupational groups in the NHS since 1973 has largely undermined this traditional belief.

The Significance of the 1973 Ancillary Workers Dispute

Whereas the national pay awards of hospital ancillary workers have tended traditionally to follow those agreed for local authority manual workers, the national dispute of hospital ancillary workers in 1973 can be stated to have directly followed from a refusal of the government to concede a pay increase similar to that agreed earlier by local authority workers and their employers. In retrospect, the dispute can be seen as a watershed in both national collective bargaining and in local workplace relationships. The active pursuit of sectional interests was not an entirely new phenomenon at the national level. For instance, some of the main organisational features of the pre-1974 Health Service were products of the initial clash between Aneurin Bevan and the doctors' representatives. Further, in 1969 the nurses had launched their 'Raise the Roof' campaign in support of their demands for higher salary scales. The uniqueness of the ancillary workers' dispute lay rather in its scale and in its public challenge to the taboo of not overtly jeopardising patient care. At a deeper level, it marked a change of direction in workplace relationships in that it presented opportunities to the ancillary workers to participate in areas of decision-making which had hitherto been the prerogative of medical and administrative staff.

Following the onset of the dispute the trade unions representing ancillary workers began to encourage, either through circumstances or by design, their union stewards to bargain with hospital managements over procedures to cope with the effects of the industrial action: the central issue of these bargaining situations being the local provision of emergency cover. Dyson in his report on the industrial action in the Leeds Region[27] points to instances where the stewards took unilateral decisions on emergency cover and it seems likely that this reflected the experiences of other Regions. Moreover, these types of decisions, together with the later steps taken to disrupt private practice constituted a direct challenge to the most powerful group within the service—the doctors. Likewise the bargaining over the emergency arrangements to cover key areas of the hotel services, e.g. laundry and catering, involved union stewards in important aspects of administrative decision-making. One implication of Dyson's report is that workplace bargaining, which was engendered by the dispute, may continue. What can also be suggested is that the dispute did not signify a complete break with the past in relation to workplace bargaining, but rather that it gave an added impetus to an awakening union consciousness amongst ancillary workers that had been developing gradually in the period immediately before 1973.

In the course of the ten years that preceded the ancillary workers' dispute, the NHS was the subject of a number of enquiries and subsequent Reports which pointed to weaknesses in the managerial arrangements of a number of health professions.[28] In 1967, the Prices and Incomes Board (PIB), in its examination of low pay amongst ancillary workers, drew attention to the need for more efficient management and the adoption of work-study techniques to combat the generally low levels of pay and productivity. The effect of these reports and PIB investigations was to encourage the introduction of industrial management techniques into the service. However, little attention at that time appears to have been given to the probable changes in workers' attitudes that could accompany the adoption of techniques such as work study. It is widely believed that payment-by-result systems may disturb the delicate balance of workplace relationships[29] and a common and not misplaced view within the Service is that this indeed was one effect of incentive bonus schemes. Thus it can be argued that the emphasis on the cash nexus, the preference for schemes based on work groups, and the creation of more inflexible demarcation lines between jobs, combined to induce subtle changes in the attitude of ancillary workers towards their jobs, which, in turn, assisted the development of workplace organisation.[30] A consequent growth in the number of union stewards was recognised by the Ancillary Staffs Council in an agreement[31] which defined their functions and their position within hospitals was further consolidated by legislation.

The complacent attitude towards local industrial relations among hospital managements which had been nurtured by the apparent predominance of Whitleyism was rudely challenged by the Conservative government's Industrial Relations Act of 1971 and its associated Code of Industrial Relations practice. The suggested obligations in the Code placed on management generally to draw up procedures that were relevant to individual establishments had immediate and unforeseen

implications for the NHS. The complexity of Whitley's represen-
tational arrangements plus a degree of bureaucratic lethargy had often
hampered speedy reactions to change. Therefore, in the absence of
specific advice on model procedures or an agreed national procedure,
hospital managements either introduced procedures unilaterally or
negotiated them directly with trade union officials. Necessarily, the
successful operation of these procedures required the involvement of
the union steward. By curious irony, therefore, legislation which was
designed to buttress the 'formal system' of British industrial relations
in the NHS acted to heighten the union consciousness of management
and worker alike and spurred on the development of workplace
organisation.

Thus the 1973 ancillary dispute broke out upon a scene, particularly in large hospitals in industrial areas, of rising expectations and
developing trade union organisation amongst ancillary workers. The
suggestion that union stewards and the active sections of the membership would be reluctant to return to their pre-dispute pattern of
acquiescent behaviour was vindicated by subsequent events. Following
the settlement of the national dispute, there were sporadic outbreaks
of industrial action over local matters in both England and Wales. The
unwillingness of ancillary workers to accept, without question, the
continued exercise of managerial prerogatives was to culminate in the
events at the Charing Cross Hospital in 1974. In July of that year, the
hospital attracted national publicity following the decision taken by
members of the ancillary staff to withdraw domestic and hotel facilities in support of their demand that the private wing be closed. The
significance of Charing Cross lies in the degree to which ancillary
workers were prepared to exercise their perceived ability to control
decision-making, to the extent of entering into tripartite negotiations
with local consultants and the Secretary of State.

Meanwhile, the continuing preoccupation of the centre with the
appropriate *methodology* for increased participation rather than with
its substance suggests that the reorganised service is still a victim of
overcentralisation in its industrial relations policies. More importantly,
as will be argued below, this preoccupation suggests that the centre
suffers from a certain lack of appreciation of the significance behind
recent developments in workplace relationships.

The Proposals for Increased Participation

'Worker Directors'

The commitment of a Labour government, returned in 1974, to the extension of industrial democracy through worker representation on company boards in the private sector was translated into Health Service terms by the Secretary of State's decision to alter the composition of health authorities. The decision was first announced in the Consultative Document, 'Democracy in the National Health Service'.[32] A subsequent Health Service Circular,[33] similarly titled 'Democracy in the National Health Service', proposed that membership of the Regional and Area health authorities should include two employee representatives in addition to the medical and nursing members. A further Consultative Paper [34] announced that the appointment of these additional 'worker directors' would be by election and invited senior managers of health authorities to comment on the proposed election arrangements. It is interesting to note, however, that while the appropriate methodology for their appointment is a matter for discussion, the central authority does not appear to have entered into a general dialogue with senior Health Service managers over the substance of participation. Moreover, although involvement in this form is exclusive to members of nationally recognised negotiating bodies, once elected, staff members will serve on health authorities in a private rather than a trade union capacity.

The concept of worker directors is largely alien to the mainstream of British industrial relations experience. While trade union officials have been appointed to the boards of nationalised industries, they have generally been selected from unions who are not primarily concerned with that particular industry and they have relinquished their union posts. They have not been required, nor have they sought, to act as workers' representatives.

In Europe, where the system of worker and trade union director is more widespread, the evidence suggests that the notion suffers from an inherent problem of obtaining a sense of either identification or commitment from the work-force.[35] Nor does it appear to have assisted the work-force in achieving a diminution of managerial control over matters of policy. However, in their recent espousal of a system of board level representation similar to that in Europe, the Trades Union Congress was clear that the inclusion of workpeople's representatives on the boards of public and private organisations was for the purpose of obtaining joint control. The TUC's [36] view of the nature of this form of participation is that it should enable the trade unions to be involved in far-reaching board-level decisions which in the past have been taken unilaterally by management. Although the Secretary of State had made the decision to introduce worker directors into the NHS at a time when the issue of industrial democracy was being examined by the Bullock Committee [37] and against the background of a heated national debate, the proposal appears to have taken little cognisance of the experience of Europe or the views expressed by the TUC.

Health Service worker directors will have to perform a difficult role. As the Consultative Paper states: 'These two extra members. . . will together with other members of their Authority be corporately responsible to the Secretary of State. . . for carrying out the functions delegated to them.' [38] The British Steel Corporation's experiment with worker directors recognised that one initial determinant of their ability to take part in board decisions was the extent to which they could cope with the concepts and techniques of industrial management. Accordingly, steps were taken, with the agreement of the unions, to ensure that the directors received the necessary training beofre they assumed their duties.[39] In Germany, those representatives who are nominated from the Works Councils to sit on Supervisory Boards will also have received, in the normal course of events, some form of training which will assist them in their roles. The question of who should be responsible for the training of worker directors is problematic. Both the trade unions and management can advance reasoned arguments to justify their respective responsibility for this function. In the Health Service, given that the representatives are expected to act in a personal capacity, management could presumably put forward a strong claim. To date, however, little consideration appears to have been given to this vital feature: an omission which has a parallel with the decision not to train representatives for the original form of joint consultation that was introduced in 1950.

The feelings of non-involvement expressed by German workers over this type of participation need to be balanced against the belief expressed in the Consultative Paper that the new health authority members 'will be aware of the view of their fellow-workers and so help to ensure that authorities are fully responsive to the importance of staff relations in all aspects of their work.' A problem which is frequently experienced by most representatives is their ability to accurately reflect the views of their constituents. Health authorities are large undertakings and the absence of report-back systems may exacerbate the problem of accurate representation, thereby further diminishing the sense of worker involvement. Thus in extreme circumstances the Service's worker directors may in fact be representing the views of only their immediate work group.

It has been suggested that the introduction of joint consultation in 1950 was not undertaken in response to a deeply felt need, but as a concession to a fashion in social thinking.[40] One conclusion that could be drawn about the Service's proposals for increased democracy is that it too is merely a concession to contemporary social trends. Whilst it is inappropriate to draw a firm conclusion at this stage, it should be recorded that many of its features which have been discussed were examined by the Donovan Commission in their deliberations over the introduction of company-level representation. As a result of their examinations, a majority of the Commission rejected this form of participation on the grounds that it was unlikely to give workers a real share in, or control over, the work of the boards that they joined.[41]

Joint Consultation and Participative Management

If worker directors offer no means to influence management decision-making, what then of joint consultation? At the time of writing, a revised system of joint consultation has still to be agreed by the General Whitley Council. Informed but unofficial management and trade union sources have referred to a number of disputes which have tended to polarise opinions between the two sides of the Council, and which have their parallel in the negotiations that preceded the introduction of the original form of joint consultation in 1950. Furthermore, in its draft form, the proposal does not appear to exhibit a major change in attitude on management's part.[42] The Circular on 'Participative Management'[43] defines it as a method of enabling more staff in the Health Service to become involved in changing for the better the way that they work. This is to be achieved by improved communications between management and staff and the establishment of joint working groups to consider operational problems. However, the decisions of these groups will not diminish the responsibilities of management. The nature of these two proposals suggests an absence of any real shift in attitude towards participation. Indeed, they both retain the firm commitment to the continued exercise of traditional managerial authority.

The desire of the centre to maintain the prerogatives of hospital managements is not here at issue; rather it is the ability of hospital managements to *exercise* their traditional control, particularly in relation to the ancillary workers.

Now, the development of workplace bargaining, although it may have far-reaching consequences for an organisation's internal industrial relations, does not necessarily lead to a decline in the regulative powers of an industry-wide agreement. The Royal Commission's analysis of the development of the 'informal system' in British industrial relations was, they noted, 'described mainly in terms of private industry, and not so much in terms of public employment'.[44] The opportunities for actual wage bargaining at the workplace are considerably diminished in the public sector: the lesser number of employers and a watchful government have largely maintained the capacity of national agreements to control earnings.

Of course, the NHS is not typical of British industry. It is financed directly from the Exchequer, and government has certain safeguards which allow for stricter control of wages than is normal in industrial organisations. In addition to the control over the appointed managerial authorities given to the Secretary of State, there are supplementary powers to issue regulations and directions. These have been used to make it an offence to pay more or less than the rate agreed in the Whitley Councils except by the express permission of the Secretary of State. The introduction of a payment-by-results system amongst ancillary workers may promote local instances of wage bargaining but the range of national controls suggests that its effects will be marginal when set against total labour costs. However, the general absence of opportunities for local wage determination does not prevent shop stewards from finding issues on which to bargain, as is demonstrated by their behaviour in nationalised industries.[45]

So the development of workplace bargaining and the growth of union stewards representing the ancillary work-force, while it seems unlikely at this stage to have dire consequences for the Health Service's national bargaining arrangements, may offer a critical challenge to any new system of consultation. The draft of the proposed new agreement on joint consultation still largely retains the essential philosophy of the 1950 system, i.e. a 'method of promoting collaboration between two or more groups which have some objectives in common'. The effect of workplace bargaining on the nature of this type of participation has received a great deal of attention.[46] As McCarthy has concluded,[47] two propositions can be advanced with reasonable certainty about the relationship between shop steward bargaining and joint consultative committees. First, stewards do not subscribe to the assumptions behind the establishment of separate machinery for so-called 'conflicting' and 'common-interest' questions. Second, consultative committees that assume a philosophy of common interest and preclude the negotiation of binding agreements must either become negotiating bodies or suffer boycott by the stewards. Yet, the NHS does not possess 'separate institutional arrangements' for negotiation and consultation and, aside from the Regional Appeals Committees whose concern is with the interpretation of the various industry-wide agreements, there are no hierarchically structured negotiating arrangements similar to those in the public sector of industry. In the absence of agreed local negotiating machinery, what then are the possible implications for the Service's proposed system of joint consultation in the light of McCarthy's two propositions?

The first implication is that the volume of bargaining in large hospitals is likely to increase; even if the issue of wages is excluded from the bargaining process there are many suitable subjects for local joint determination. The second implication is that in the absence of local bargaining arrangements, hospital managements may have to create some form of unofficial machinery in which joint determination can take place. The third implication is that the ancillary workers' stewards will turn to the proposed consultative committees in an endeavour to change their character to include aspects of negotiations. A further and longer-term implication relates to the limited opportunities within hospitals for wage bargaining. It is a common assumption that shop stewards are essentially a product of private industry and that they achieved prominence due to the measure of control they were able to exert over the determination of their members' earnings. Almost invariably the reality is more complex. However, behind the common assumption there is a grain of truth, i.e. in circumstances where there was a discretionary element over wage fixing, stewards quite naturally were drawn into a system of wage bargaining. In consequence, they were less concerned to participate in other aspects of management decision-making, e.g. take-overs and mergers, investment policy, manpower planning and recruitment. It is only very recently that unions have sought legal involvement in these issues. In the Health Service, stewards may seek a similar extension of control in decisions over the closure and rationalisation of hospitals and staff redundancy.

The implications of McCarthy's propositions for the new form of Health Service joint consultation suggest that the proposals for participative management will be unacceptable to organised groups of ancillary workers. Its underlying rationale is that the Service is a unitary organisation [48] in which its staff are striving to achieve a common goal and the 'care of the patient' is a commonly declared goal of all occupational groups. However, the ancillary workers' dispute and the subsequent industrial action taken by most groups up to the time of writing demonstrates that the superordinate goal may, on occasions, be neglected in the pursuit of short-term sectional interests. Indeed, it may never have had any real presence except in the minds of Health Service management, who mistakenly ascribed the absence of industrial conflict to the force of the common objective rather than to the low level of workplace organisation. The DHSS's espousal of it in the document on participative management and the belief that staff will want to be involved in changing their methods of work is therefore open to question. Staff who are not involved in workplace bargaining may welcome it as an opportunity to influence some aspects of their immediate job environment. However, a system of management, the essence of which is the recognition of 'the needs of people at work and, through involvement, to give a level of job satisfaction',[49] but which is equally concerned not to redefine the responsibilities of management, may be viewed with suspicion by those groups of workers who are concerned to achieve genuine participation. The experience of workplace bargaining in industry suggests that in general unionised workers are prepared to accept changes in work practices if management is prepared to concede either that the changes are the subject of bargaining or that the work-force receives a proportion of the projected savings. It remains to be seen how far ancillary workers will follow the example of their industrial counterparts.

The extent to which hospital managements could effectively resist these types of demands is also a matter for conjecture. The 1973 dispute shook the confidence of some hospital managements and confirmed the ability of others.[50] However, hospital managements suffer from a number of disabilities which affect their capacity to withstand persistent pressure from stewards to increase the subjects for joint determination. The first, and more important, disability arises from the nature of the Service's business: the need to provide patients with the necessary medical and hotel facilities denies to managers, at each organisational level within the Service, the use of many of the sanctions which are employed by industrial management in conflict situations. Indeed the organisation of the Service itself may act as a disability: the sense of remoteness which seems to pervade the relationship between the centre and the remainder of the Service may be just as keenly felt in the relationships between District, Area and Region; and the separate managerial hierarchies within the different occupational groups can militate against the establishment of consistent industrial relations policies and practices at the District level. Finally, neither the formal collective bargaining machinery nor the reorganised structure were designed to encompass a system of workplace bargaining. In consequence, hospital managements may frequently, without central guidance, face industrial action over issues which are outside their power to settle. In these circumstances their capacity to exercise their traditional authority must be in doubt.

Conclusions

This paper has attempted to demonstrate that the traditional forms of Health Service participation possessed a dominant underlying philosophy, the regulation of actual earnings and the preservation of the prerogatives of hospital management, and that the proposals for increased participation retain this basic commitment to managerial control. The extent to which the industrial relations experiences of British and European industry have been ignored by these proposals suggests that the central decision-makers have failed to appreciate the significance of the development of workplace organisation amongst ancillary workers. This development suggests that ancillary workers will seek forms of participation which will allow them to exercise a degree of control over management decisions. Their desire for genuine participation may mean that the present proposals will prove unacceptable. Thus the appointment of worker directors in a personal capacity does not appear to be an adequate means of involving the work-force. Joint consultation and participative management, in their present forms, may be equally unsuccessful; their nature may either then be changed to encompass workplace bargaining, or, following their introduction, they may merely come to operate in impotent isolation from the more informal vehicles of worker participation.

Notes

1. Department of Health and Social Security, *Health and Personal Social Services Statistics, 1974,* HMSO, London, 1975.
2. J. P. R. French, Jnr., J. Israel and D. As, 'An experiment on participation in a Norwegian factory', *Human Relations,* Vol. 13, 1960.
3. K. F. Walker, 'Workers' Participation in Management: Concepts and Reality', *Industrial Relations and the Wider Society,* B. Barrett, E. Rhodes and J. Beishon (eds.), Collier Macmillan, London, 1975.
4. A. S. Tannenbaum, *Social Psychology of the Work Organisation,* Tavistock Publications, London, 1966, p.83.
5. P. Bachrach and Morton S. Baratz, *Power and Poverty: Theory and Practice,* Oxford University Press, New York, 1970, p.8.
6. C. J. Lammers, 'Power and participation in decision making in formal organisations', *American Journal of Sociology,* Vol. 73, No. 2, 1967.

7. *Royal Commission on Trade Unions and Employers' Associations* (Cmnd. 3623), HMSO, London, 1968—commonly referred to as the 'Donovan Report'.

8. In October 1916, following a sequence of unofficial strikes that were associated with the Shop Steward Movement, the government set up a Committee on the Relations between Employers and Employed, under the chairmanship of J. H. Whitley, MP, who at the time was the Deputy Speaker of the House of Commons. The recommendations contained in the five reports submitted by the Committee have played an important role in the extension and formation of joint negotiating machinery in Britain since that time.

9. The collective bargaining arrangements of the National Health Service consist of a General Whitley Council made up of management representatives drawn from the Department of Health and Social Security, the Scottish Home and Health Department, Regional Health Authorities, and other levels of management. The staff representatives are drawn from recognised trade unions and professional associations who have places on the ten Functional Councils. The main function of the General Council is to negotiate aspects of remuneration and conditions of service which are common to all Health Service staff. The ten Functional Councils are also joint bodies and negotiate on the remuneration and conditions of service which are particular to the various occupational groups, namely Ambulance; Administrative and Clerical; Ancillary; Dental; Medical; Nurses and Midwives; Optical; Pharmaceutical; Professional and Technical 'A' and 'B'.

10. See for instance, H. A. Clegg and T. E. Chester, *Wage Policy and the Health Service,* Basil Blackwell, Oxford, 1957, pp.77-9. Also in 1957, a pay increase for administrative and clerical staff was agreed against the Government's wishes and subsequently vetoed by the Minister of Health, Derek Walker-Smith, thus highlighting the limits to the power of the staff side.

11. H. A Clegg and T. E. Chester, op. cit., p.91.

12. A. W. Miles and Duncan Smith, *Joint Consultation: Defeat or Opportunity?,* King's Fund, London, 1969, p.16.

13. For example, in 1974, a separate Inquiry under Lord Halsbury was established to examine the pay of nurses and midwives. Its reference was subsequently widened to include certain professional and technical groups.

14. Rudolf Klein, 'Policy Problems and Policy Perceptions in the National Health Service', *Policy and Politics,* Vol. 2, No. 3, 1974.

15. Harry Eckstein, *Pressure Group Politics; the case of the British Medical*

16. H. A. Clegg and T. E. Chester, op. cit., p.120.

17. National Board for Prices and Incomes, *Report No. 29: the pay and conditions of manual workers in Local Authorities, the National Health Service, Gas and Water Supply,* HMSO, London, 1967.

18. Subsequently referred to in the Report of the Royal Commission on Trade Unions and Employers' Associations, op. cit., p.12.

19. *General Whitley Council: Conditions of Service,* Whitley Councils of the Health Services (Great Britain), London, 1968, Section XXIV, p.39.

20. R. O. Clarke, D. J. Fatchett and B. C. Roberts, *Workers Participation in Management in Britain,* Heinemann, London, 1972, pp.9-10.

21. *General Whitley Council: Conditions of Service,* op. cit., p.36.

22. *General Whitley Council: Conditions of Service,* op. cit., p.39.

23. W. E. J. McCarthy, 'The Role of Shop Stewards in British Industrial Relations', *Royal Commission on Trade Unions and Employers' Associations Research Paper No. 1,* HMSO, London, 1966, p.36.

24. For an authoritative report of this period, see A. W. Miles and Duncan Smith, op. cit.

25. *Report of the Ministry of Health, 1952* (Cmnd. 8933), HMSO, London, 1953, p.111.
26. D. High, A. McDowell, R. Meara and J. Sharpley, 'Hospitals and Industrial Relations', *British Hospital Journal and Social Science Review*, Vol. 82, No.2, 1972.
27. R. F. Dyson, *Ancillary Staff Industrial Action, Spring, 1973*, Leeds Regional Hospital Board, Leeds, 1974, p.5.
28. For example: *Report of the Committee on Senior Nursing Structure*, (Salmon Report), HMSO, London, 1966; *Report of the Working Party on the Hospital Pharmaceutical Service* (Noel-Hall Report), HMSO, London, 1970; *Report of Committee on Hospital, Scientific and Technical Services* (Zuckerman Report), HMSO, London, 1968.
29. The following are some of the sources that have commented on the effects on workplace relationships of payment-by-results systems: National Board for Prices and Incomes, *Report No. 65: Payment by Results Systems*, HMSO, London, 1968; Royal Commission on Trade Unions and Employers' Associations, op. cit.; Alan Fox, *Beyond Contract: Work, Power and Trust Relations*, Faber and Faber, London, 1974.
30. S. J. Dimmock and D. Farnham, 'Working with Whitley in today's NHS', *Personnel Management*, January 1975.
31. *Ancillary Staff Council: Rates of Pay, Conditions of Service*, Whitley Councils for Health Services, London, 1972, Part IX.
32. Department of Health and Social Security, *Democracy in the National Health Service*, HMSO, London, 1974.
33. *Democracy in the National Health Service*, HSC(IS)194, DHSS, London, September 1975.
34. *Democracy in the National Health Service: Election of Staff Members of Authorities, Ref. N/H223/2*, DHSS, London, January 1976.
35. For example, F. Furstenberg, 'Workers' Participation in Management in the Federal Republic of Germany', *International Institute for Labour Studies*, Bulletin 6, 1969, has shown that many workers were unaware of either the introduction or the meaning of the system of codetermination in their firms. F. E. Emery and E. Thorsrud, *Form and Content in Industrial Democracy*, Tavistock Publications, London, 1969, p.83, also comment on the inability of worker directors to make an impact on the working lives of their constituents.
36. Trades Union Congress, *Industrial Democracy: Interim Report*, Trades Union Congress, London, 1973.
37. Bullock Committee of Inquiry on Industrial Democracy appointed in 1975, and due to report in 1977.
38. *Democracy in the National Health Service*, Ref. N/H223/2, op. cit., p.1.
39. P. Brannen, E. Batstone and D. Fatchett, *The Worker Directors*, Hutchinson, London, 1976.
40. A. W. Miles and Duncan Smith, op. cit., p.41.
41. Royal Commission on Trade Unions and Employers' Associations, op. cit., pp.257-9.
42. The author has had the opportunity to study the management-side draft.
43. Department of Health and Social Security, *Health Services Development: Participative Management*, HC(76)44, London, September 1976.
44. Royal Commission on Trade Unions and Employers' Associations, op. cit., p.36.
45. W. E. J. McCarthy, op. cit., p.12.
46. See for example: H. A. Clegg, *A New Approach to Industrial Democracy*, Blackwell, Oxford, 1960; W. H. Scott, *Coal and Conflict: A Study of Indus-*

rial Relations at Collieries, Liverpool University Press, 1963; A. I. Marsh and E. Coker, 'Shop Steward Organisation in Engineering', *British Journal of Industrial Relations,* Vol. 1, No. 2, 1973.

47. W. E. J. McCarthy, op. cit. '
48. For a discussion of the implications of management's view of the unitary nature of organisations, see Alan Fox, *Royal Commission on Trade Unions and Employers' Associations, Research Paper No. 3: Industrial Sociology and Industrial Relations,* HMSO, 1966. And for a self-criticism of his former views, see Alan Fox, 'A Social Critique of Pluralist Ideology', in J. Child (ed.), *Man and Organisation,* George Allen and Unwin, London, 1973.
49. C. W. Dickinson and I. R. Hodgetts, 'Participation in Practice', *Health and Social Services Journal,* 18 October 1975, p.2338.
50. R. F. Dyson, op. cit.

7 HEALTH ADMINISTRATION AND THE JAUNDICE OF REORGANISATION

J. Crossley Sunderland

At a time of seemingly growing public discontent with bureaucracy and public officials, the administrator in the National Health Service is identified with the management system which has generated much of the discontent about the Service, despite the many reservations he increasingly shares with its critics. He has come to be seen as the personification of the system and hence as the appropriate target for (and, paradoxically, respondent to) criticism about it.

The purpose of this essay therefore is to look at the issues from the administrator's perspective and to show how the administrator is constrained by the management system to as great an extent as are any of the other professionals working within the NHS. The essay has four main sections. The first examines some of the key concepts in the history of administration in the NHS from the early fifties to the present day and looks, *inter alia,* at the creation of functional management posts; the case for the appointment of a chief executive officer; the role of the hospital secretary; Health Service team management and the emphasis of the seventies on management generally. Secondly, the role of the administrator in the new 'political' arena is examined. The complex arrangements for scrutiny and consultation are considered and their effect on the administrator who thus has a delicate balance of influences to maintain. Thirdly, the role of the administrator at the level of institutional management is examined together with the practical problems discovered in trying to apply certain theories of management[1] which appear appropriate in the health field. In conclusion, consideration is given to a support-gap between the 'political' and institutional levels of administration and the view is expressed that a different style of support to that which currently holds good, is crucial if administration of hospitals is not to fall below the high standard which had been achieved by the time of NHS reorganisation.

Historical Perspective

The starting point for a consideration of administration in the NHS is the Bradbeer Report.[2] This committee saw hospital administration as being split into medical, nursing and lay administration and, whilst recognising that there were distinct duties for each of the three, emphasised the need to work together as a team. It was further stressed that neither the medical nor nursing administrator should, as a rule, do work which a layman could do equally well. For the efficient administration of the hospital service the committee recommended one chief administrative officer at Hospital Management Committee level, who would co-ordinate the work of all departments and keep them under continuous review. Only at hospital level was tripartism deemed appropriate and feasible. The committee also considered the introduction of specialist posts in finance and supply and saw this as a logical conclusion to the integration of groups of hospitals into larger administrative units. It was felt that as a general rule all principal officers at group level should be responsible to the governing body through the chief administrative officer, the Group Secretary. Some difficulty was found in reconciling the need to avoid undue administrative costs with the principle of dividing responsibility for spending public funds and responsibility for accounting for them between more than one officer. Somewhat inconclusively, the committee took the view that on occasion the combination of the posts of secretary, finance officer and supply officer might be appropriate, but that generally the two former posts, at least, should remain separate. Noel Hall,[3] while pointing to difficulties arising from the wide variety of posts carrying the title hospital secretary, none the less advocated as much delegation to that officer as possible. Continuing the tripartite analysis of Bradbeer,[4] this report regarded the hospital secretary as the general manager, but with specific duties in the same way as those accorded to his nursing and medical administrative colleagues. The hospital secretary was to be regarded as one of the key support officers to the group secretary on matters of policy. Farquharson-Lang[5] saw a tendency in the sphere of non-medical administration towards a concentration of secretarial functions at the expense of planning and management. In their recommendations this Scottish committee attempted to reduce the secretarial burden by changing the role of member-Boards, leaving the chief officers more time to deal with management, which in turn implied a new role for them. It was felt that hospital Boards of Management underestimated the importance of administration when assessing their staffing needs, falling prey to the more emotional demands for medical and nursing requirements in a Service where patient welfare is the prime objective. The committee looked carefully at the arguments for and against the appointment of a chief executive officer and while much of the evidence submitted to them indicated a theoretical desire for such an appointment, in practice the view was expressed that multipartite administration had existed too long to be effectively changed. None the less, on balance the advantages of a single channel of administration were endorsed and the proposal made that a chief executive post be established at each type of Board. This report thus anticipated one of the reorganisation debates, since the architects of the 'Management Arrangements for the reorganised NHS'[6] were also to wrestle with the idea of recommending a chief officer appointment, only to reach a different conclusion, and interestingly the Farquharson-Lang proposal was never implemented.

It was during this time, the sixties, that the professions of finance, supply, nursing and technology were also examining their own administrative structures and were developing pyramidal career structures which demanded parity of status if they were to be workable. Team management was thus rapidly becoming a political reality. Consensus management was an inevitable response, albeit compromise, in the face of pressure from vested interests. Yet, paradoxically the climate of the seventies and of the immediate pre-reorganisation period emphasised managerial skill and ability and sought to elevate the administrator as a major instrument in developing a more rational, more effective and more efficient Health Service. The NHS Reorganisation Consultative Document[7] wished to establish an atmosphere based on 'effective management'. However, as will be argued in this essay, it is a pledge which is in danger of causing jaundice in that the management arrangements that emerged after expert study may progressively render the administrator less rather than more effective.

The Administrator as 'Politician'

Administration in the NHS can be viewed as operating at two levels. There is a policy and strategy level which, in the context of the many consultative and administrative constraints put upon it, seeks to ensure not only that a service is provided, but that the optimum service is provided and that improvements are facilitated. And, complementary to this, there is an institutional level at which the patient receives service.

In considering the administrator who is involved in the policy and (political) arena, the focus is on the Area Administrators, District Administrators and their immediate support staff, since it is they who have had to respond to pressures on and in an NHS which has, for some time and increasingly in recent years, become the stage on which a wide variety of groups and organisations have demonstrated their political influence within the public sector.[8] The practical constraints on administration at this level as a result of political complications manifest themselves in a number of ways. In the first place, the administrator is now faced with a number of new external relationships which he has either not met before or encountered only to a limited degree. Secondly, as indicated in the report undertaken by a Working Party of the Association of Chief Administrators of Health Authorities (ACAHA) his problems are being posed in terms of

> uncertainties about relationships, about functions and above all, about responsibilities. In the absence of clear objectives and faced with a completely new structure, other problems concerned with the mere performance of tasks have become pre-eminent. The need to survive in, or despite, the new system.[9]

Thirdly, and on a broad scale, the NHS is itself becoming the subject of increasingly complicated arrangements for scrutiny. This is, to a degree, understandable in a Service which is readily identified as publicly financed and which is expected to attain extremely high standards. However, it can and does impose further constraints on administrative practice.

Key stages in the development of this scrutiny have been: the admission of the press and public to meetings of health authorities,[10] the increasing number of committees of enquiry and the establishment of the (now) Health Advisory Service,[11] the setting up of the Office of the Health Service Commissioner,[12] the Davies Report[13] on hospital complaints procedures; the complex arrangements in the reorganised National Health Service for consultative and advisory machinery; the establishment of Community Health Councils,[14] and most recently, the decision to establish a Royal Commission.

Central to the issue of scrutiny is the relationship between appointed members of health authorities and the officers—whether or not the former hold executive or representative authority. The relationship was considered in detail by Farquharson-Lang,[15] which was extremely critical of Boards which intervened in the details of administration and felt that once a decision had been taken, it ought to have been framed in such a manner that officers could proceed to act upon it without further reference to the membership. Quite simply, Farquharson-Lang[16] took the view that it was the role of the member that should be circumscribed, rather than that of the officer, in order to provide an effective working arrangement.

In the Consultative Document,[17] Sir Keith Joseph envisaged a style of membership which brought something intrinsically new to the Service—management expertise from other spheres of business and administration. The character of the new membership was inclined to taking the lead. The situation was compounded by the absence of any countervailing influence in the early days of the reorganised Service. Officers had not yet been appointed and chairmen in particular became the personification of the Authority. As the 'Appointed Day' drew nearer, and indeed in the immediate post period, it must have often proved difficult to wean chairmen away from this acquisition of direct influence, particularly as they were being remunerated for their efforts. In contrast, Farquharson-Lang,[18] alert to the dangers that a chairman might be tempted to become the managing director and to take over responsibilities which should properly fall upon officers, had taken the view that the appointment of a chief executive officer would be the principle means of reducing the extent to which a chairman would need to be called in to resolve particular issues. NHS reorganisation was to see a different picture emerge.

In the new NHS order, the phenomenon of an active rather than passive chairman and a membership that aspires to be a decision-making body makes access to the Authority a matter of central concern to senior officers. A principle source of contention between the District and Area Administration is that, while the Area Administrator is the official link between the Authority and its officers, the link between the District Administrator and the Authority members, and in particular the chairman, is more tenuous. The attendance of all appropriate senior officers at meetings of the Authority serves several purposes; it enables the Authority to have the specialised advice of its officers to bear directly on the problems being discussed, it keeps officers in touch with policy debates and the way their work is affected, and it promotes a more effective dialogue between officer and member. Since 1974 the issue has assumed major importance for the District Management Team (DMT). Being theoretically directly accountable to the Authority, they have come to regard lack of access to the membership in general, and the chairman in particular, as being not far removed from saying that they are to work through the Area Team of Officers and that a line relationship exists between the teams, in direct contradiction of their official parity of status within the Authority. The consequence is conflict, whereas the system assumes co-operation.

In 1974 the change of government, whilst it produced a promise not to introduce early changes to the structure of the reorganised NHS, did produce an attempt to change the character of the membership. In 'Democracy in the National Health Service'[19] three major changes were envisaged: an increase to one-third for local authority membership on health authorities (the Statutory Instrument[20] to effect this has since been laid); representation for Community Health Council members on health authorities (this has, in fact, resulted in the agreement whereby a Community Health Council spokesman shall have speaking, but not voting, rights at health authority meetings) and representation for trade union members on health authorities.

The relationship between appointed members and administrators has also changed now that the number of public representatives involved has increased. The Area or District Administrator now deals additionally with members of Family Practitioner Committees, Joint Consultative Committees and Community Health Councils. The situation of the Family Practitioner Committee raises particular difficulties for the Area Administrator, who is not really involved at all with this separate body of members. The ACAHA Report has suggested that 'the Department's influence is no longer directed towards increasingly integrating Family Practitioner Committee services with the remainder, and rather the reverse is occurring.'[21]

The report points to the gradual establishment of independence by Family Practitioner Committees, and suggests that there are divided loyalties for Administrators (Family Practitioner Services). The position is thus one in which, having been challenged to take up the wider responsibilities of an integrated service, Area Administrators are now finding that some policy decisions in the field of primary care cannot always be brought to the attention of the Area Health Authority.

The establishment of Joint Consultative Committees, as part of the statutory arrangements for collaboration with local government, and the local authority presence in the Area Health Authority membership has brought the administrator and the elected Councillor into close contact. Because the local government representatives sit on the Joint Consultative Committees as locally elected officials and are therefore in many cases more politically vunerable than their nationally and regionally selected health authority counterparts, they are thus often keen to either make an immediate impact in order to demonstrate their effectiveness or to refrain from committing themselves until the odds are favourable. Rightly or wrongly, it is in dealing with this style of membership that the former hospital administrator finds his ability to influence and to take charge is more inhibited than in years gone by.

The ACAHA report also provides an account of the way in which

administrators have greeted the arrival of the Community Health Council member and it records that Community Health Councils are tending
'to see themselves as part of management, exerting power without
responsibility',[22] and this trend is seen as more significant with the
arrangements whereby the Community Health Councils are able to send
a spokesman to the meetings of the Area Health Authority, when in
some authorities members of the District Management Team are not
themselves in attendance. It is a fairly obvious argument to claim parity,
in that at least one representative of the District Management Team
ought to be present to put the team's views at meetings of the Authority,
in so far as these may conflict with the views which are being advanced
by the Community Health Council spokesman. In such circumstances
the threat as seen by the administrator (or indeed the District Management Team) is that of Community Health Councils beginning to act as
'House Committees', or as the legitimate spokesman for their districts.
The intriguing converse is that some administrators have found in the
Community Health Council a useful ally and a particular means of
channelling dissatisfaction with political decisions through regular and
irregular paths back to source.

The change in relationships introduced into the administrator's
pattern of work is also marked by his being joined by nursing, financial and clinical colleagues in a management team. Whatever the
merits of the leadership style of the administrator may have been in
the past, he inevitably now has less of his own way. dealing on (more)
equal terms with other professionals who have also, more than likely,
been in charge of their own organisations. Some administrators have
eschewed the role of chairman in an attempt to demonstrate their
adaptability to the democracy of the team (and some have fallen back
on the fact that the administrator is the official co-ordinator and
channel of communication). Some teams have not appointed chairmen at all. Whatever the team structure, after so many years of solo
practice, consensus is not something that comes naturally to the individuals who make it up.

As indicated earlier, the relationship *between* teams based at the
different tiers still shows signs of stress. One of the more novel features
of the post-reorganisation management arrangements has been the device
of monitoring to counter the tendency to disorganisation when staff are
not in a hierarchical relationship. Monitoring can be summed up as the
right and duty to observe and comment on the performance of
colleagues, who might in other organisational circumstances be a subordinate, but ordinarily not the right to instruct them to take corrective

action. The full flowering of the monitoring relationship is seen in the status of the Area and District officer teams, who, being directly responsible to the same authority, are best distinguished by their respective roles of monitors and monitored. The monitors seem to be unsure as to their role and the monitored are not clear how they are meant to react. There do not yet appear to be any ground rules in relation to monitoring, certainly norms in the administration field are few and far between by which to monitor and sanctions which can be applied at the discretion of the monitors appear either elusive or non-existent.

Perhaps the most obvious practical constraint to administrative efficiency which is a product of the political backcloth to the NHS is in the field of industrial relations, where often a localised protest about a national policy seriously affects the administrator who is, of course, in no position to satisfy the demands of the protestors. The reorganisation of the NHS was greeted by a spate of industrial action and it is probably the case that, in the language of the historian, reorganisation was the occasion but not the cause.[23] The background of inflation and the wages spiral which meant the disappearance of countless development programmes within the NHS and the non-implementation of proper management arrangements for many of the professions immediately following reorganisation precipitated many trade unions and professional organisations to demonstrate their dissatisfaction—knowing that in the Health Service they were sure of drawing attention to the point they were trying to make.

It is a popular belief, particularly among health workers, that the administrators suffered less in the change to the reorganised NHS than did other groups of staff, given their opportunities for dramatic promotion. Or, if they did suffer, by virtue of being the managers of the change, the administrators were dealt with first in the reallocation of personnel and therefore had more time to recover from the trauma. It is the frequency with which this type of criticism of administrators is publicly aired that makes it difficult for their problems to be viewed sympathetically. Clearly the administrators always have had a continuity role in the NHS, and so it was only natural that they should take this on in respect of reorganisation and manage the change as well as be a part of it.[24] That the NHS survived the transition is arguably an indication of how well the administrators succeeded in managing the change. Even if it had not been dealt with first, the administrative profession would still have taken it upon itself to manage the change, rather than be a disruptive influence in the period of change-over.

The administrators are currently fond of reminding the other professionals that administration is, as yet, the only professional group which has not resorted to withdrawal of services in order to ensure that a point of view is drawn to wider attention. Even so, the Institute of Health Service Administrators has recently considered whether it should respond to requests for solidarity from other professional associations and trade unions who are in dispute, when this will involve the disruption of health services. This whole question is crucial to the continuity role which is expected of administrators. It would be impossible for them to make arrangements to ensure services in a situation where there had been withdrawal of labour by a particular group if, on a previous occasion, they had similarly withdrawn their services (and thus achieved a disruption which was far more effective in that no one had tried to allay its effects). In order not to be compromised in future situations, the administrator thus forgoes the now universally accepted basic right of other employees of withdrawing labour to influence the employer.

It can be argued that the administrator received little or no help from the other professions in facilitating the reorganisation of the NHS, indeed the latter appeared only too keen not to be seen to be tagged with the old-fashioned label of devotion to the Service and concentrated instead on delaying tactics and criticisms. Yet there is an extent to which the industrial unrest that heralded reorganisation of the NHS can be seen as an almost inevitable reflection of declining staff morale, and not as just destruction tactics by those professions concerned. The problem lay in the speed with which reorganisation took place. The principle of coterminous boundaries with local authorities committed the NHS to a timetable which finished on 1 April 1974 along with local government reorganisation, which left very little time in which to plan the change. However, as the industrial unrest has showed only small signs of abating in the post-reorganisation period, it is not implausible to take the view that many of the professions did not really want the new NHS to work and were happy to sit back and to criticise under the umbrella of poor industrial relations. It is a paradox in the administration of the Health Service that whilst making a challenge to the relevance of the administrator's role, other professions expect the administrator to continue to be responsible for finding organisational solutions in conditions of relative instability and industrial unrest. Thus, the situation is one in which those professions who challenge the administrator in open confrontation by taking industrial action are the same professions who look first for administrative support when their own working arrangements are interfered with by a dispute. The past few years are littered with disruptive action by groups of staff and it would be easy for the administrator to see himself as being isolated in a supportive role in the face of continual industrial dispute and disenchantment. It would also be easy for him to be self-congratulatory on the grounds that at least he has tried to make reorganisation operative. There is now a danger, however, that coping with a surfeit of industrial action may lead to a situation where the administrator feels enough is enough. There must come a time when supporting a conflict-ridden organisation is no longer something the administrator is prepared to do alone, and then the Service stands in danger.

Many of the problems discussed in this section also concern the administrators involved in institutional management, to whose problems this essay now turns, but first the argument so far should be summarised. The senior administrator is operating in a political arena, which is a new and difficult situation, certainly for the former hospital administrator whose previous environment, in retrospect, must appear a stable, tranquil and ordered organisation. However, these administrators are aware of this essential change and are making efforts to adapt themselves, whatever reservations they might have. Their ability to change, and therefore to continue to serve their authorities, their colleagues and the public in a vital role, hinges much more than has been realised on a far greater sense of understanding, particularly from colleagues in other professions. The challenge to make reorganisation work is really to them, not to the administrator.

The Administrator as Manager

A distinction has already been drawn between matters of policy and strategy and the direct provision of services; it is the administrators who are involved with this provision, the sector and unit, and in particular institutional administrators,[25] who now become the subject of examination. As with the 'political' arena, the debate centres around a conflict between theory and practice. It will be evident that there is a continuum which gives total authority to professionals at one extreme and to administrators or line managers at the other. While in the author's view theory supports the case for the line manager having major authority, with the functional professional in support, functional management had become such a well-established concept in the NHS, that a compromise offer of two alternative structures was made for the post-1974 arrangements.

The options offered for institutional administrators were those of management or co-ordination. They appear several times in the 'Management Arrangements for the Reorganised NHS', as in the following instance:

> Two basic alternative organisation patterns are possible for
> institutional services within Districts. Under the first alternative, the
> Sector Administrator manages all the support staff and is responsible
> for their budgets. Under the second, functional managers at District,
> e.g. catering and laundry managers, are responsible for the different
> services, and although they outpost staff to the sector, they remain
> responsible for the budget. Outposted staff, in this case, are subject
> to the monitoring and co-ordinating authority of the Sector
> Administrator.[26]

The theoretical patterns which these two alternatives allow can be
illustrated diagramatically. The problem of functional management is
that of two superiors and, therefore, two flows of influence—line
responsibility and advisory responsibility—to the one activity (see
Figure 1). Now, the combination implied by the first alternative gives

---

Figure 1: Division of Task Between Two Superiors

advisory/professional responsibility   line responsibility

                                    administrative
                                         task
        ('how')   box   ('what' and 'when')

---

the line responsibility to the local lay administrator and the advisory
powers to the appropriate functional manager (see Figure 2). More

---

Figure 2: Dual Influence

professional functional manager   administrator as line man-
with advisory powers   ager, committing resources
                                    administrative and holding the budget
                                         task
        ('how')   box   ('what' and 'when')

---

often, however, the pattern that has emerged is for the second alternative in which the line responsibility falls to the functional manager
whereas the advisory and co-ordinating powers fall to the lay
administrator (see Figure 3). Thus, under this option, local staff are
outposted and then directly managed by the functional professional
who, as a budget-holder, commits resources. He also has executive

Figure 3: Outposting

professional functional manager as line manager	administrative task box	administrator as co-ordinator
('what' and 'how')		('when')

authority in terms of goals. With option one the administrator faces a situation in which the service unit is always able to run for cover to a professional superior. Whilst the administrator does not find this an arrangement to be applauded, it is to him infinitely more workable than option two, where he faces considerable difficulty in co-ordinating and monitoring professional heads of departments who, installed as *line managers,* are unlikely to seek or accept lay advice.

Line-staff relations can always be a source of problems, but they have been compounded in the NHS by a drift into functional management which brings out conflict between the local administrator-line manager, local staff units and headquarters staff units at the various tiers of the Service.

The drift into functional management has been a consequence of the perceived need, in the past, to improve recruitment to the NHS, which meant competing with private sector salaries. To justify high salaries pyramidal career structures were devised and to justify the structures functional management theory was cited and invoked. Thus, although born out of a sequence of official reports relating to particular occupational groups as different as nurses, supplies officers, pharmacists and scientific officers,[27] functional management was promoted as a separately inspired theory. It could then be used to provide the rationalisation for decisions that were really already taken on quite different (economic) grounds. The precedent of each profession to its own career structure was set by these reports and the pattern became one of increasing salaries by adding yet wider parameters of management to the top of the career structure. Reorganisation provided the perfect opportunity. Whereas earlier it had been necessary to create artificial area structures,[28] tiers were now presented to be tagged with the appropriate post, regardless of any manpower plan.[29] Much of the pressure has, of course, been brought to bear by the trade unions and professional staff organisations, but they can hardly be blamed for looking after their own. Bradbeer made an early observation:

The introduction of the grouping system into the hospital service has put the senior lay administrator of the individual hospital, the sub-unit of the group, into a position which is in many ways puzzling and to some extent disputed.[30]

The King's Fund submission to the Bradbeer Committee suggested that

the development of a series of departments at group headquarters might subtract from the local unit administrator so many of his responsibilities as to make his post of but little account. . . He [the group administrator] should delegate as much responsibility and authority for everyday running to his unit administrators as is consistent with adequate supervision.[31]

Further, in considering the relationship between the unit hospital administrator and departmental heads in the hospital, it was suggested that where departmental organisations existed, for example in finance, supply, catering and engineering, the departmental heads should be responsible to the local administrator rather than to the professional officer at group headquarters, even though in the course of their everyday work the departmental heads often would deal direct with those group officers.

Bradbeer[32] weighed both the advantages and the disadvantages of a functionally managed hospital group and inclined to the view that the unit hospital administrator should have overall control lest the unit should become unduly fragmented.

Although as early as 1954 the memorandum of evidence to Bradbeer[33] from the (then) Institute of Hospital Administrators made mention of 'necessary co-ordination', 'changed position' and 'more restricted responsibility', the Institute's earlier report[34] on the administration of the hospital service had emphasised that the administrative officer in charge of the individual general hospital should be in *overall* charge (subject to the higher authority of the group secretary) and that departmental officers should be responsible to him. Additionally, instructions from various group departmental heads in matters within their technical competence were to be transmitted through the local administrator.

A more recent report, prepared by a joint working party of various professional associations representing administrators,[35] addresses itself to the recognition of the administrator's co-ordinating responsibility, simultaneous with a loosening of his involvement in daily departmental management. It documents the rapid decline in the authority of the unit

administrator since Bradbeer [36] and is firm in its view that there should
be an overall manager at local level. It argues for an administrator who
can 'evaluate the effect of change, who is accessible to both staff and
patients, and who will always be available for advice and guidance'. [37]
Observe that the image created here is of a negative influence waiting to
be consulted, rather than of a manager imposing his influence on a situation. As the influence of the locally based administrator has declined in
the face of both growing functionalism and the multiplying tiers of
administration, there has been a tendency on the part of commentators
and practitioners alike to respond by treating the *de facto* position of
the administrator as if it were his correct role:

> We are unanimously of the opinion that new management develop-
> ments (including functional management) have increased rather than
> decreased the responsibilities of the unit administrator. There is now
> a great opportunity and indeed, a requirement, for him to become
> involved and to exercise influence by virtue of his monitoring and co-
> ordinating role. [38]

The report comments upon the career patterns followed by administrators and places much importance on the experience gained in
institutional management as being a suitable preparation for future posts
of high rank, even a prerequisite for them. Paradoxically, however, the
system of institutional management which it advocates will not provide
that experience which is necessary preparation for participation in a
management team, for it cannot afford the opportunity for making
decisions.

The alternatives of management or co-ordination offered in 'Management Arrangements' [39] are not overtly acknowledged in the Working
Party's report which instead concentrates its attention on co-ordination
at the expense of authority:

> In many of the cases where there has been difficulty in developing
> the right kind of relationship between the administrators and func-
> tional managers, this has been in part due to the inability of the
> administrator to recognise his role as co-ordinator and enabler rather
> than his former responsibility for the day-to-day management of
> departments traditionally linked with administration, for example,
> catering, domestic, portering, etc. [40]

To understate the point, this is a somewhat unexpected conclusion for practising administrators to draw. By focusing on the alleged 'inability' of administrators, it implies that they lack sensitivity to local issues and need to be told to acquire it. Common sense suggests otherwise: that such sensitivity is to be found in lay administrators with their overview of hospital situations, but not in the functional managers with their circumscribed duties. This prompts the question whether it is their collective jaundice with reorganisation in practice that has led the Joint Working Party to ignore the option between management and co-ordination? It is only in the appendices of the report that reference is made to published guidance on the responsibility of sector administrators for managing or co-ordinating. It is certainly the case that the subsequent government circular[41] appears to have watered down the original scope of the management option revealed in 'Management Arrangements'.[42] The circular states that the sector administrator will manage some staff providing administrative support services, co-ordinate others and co-ordinate the interaction of the different managerial systems; 'it is not his duty to co-ordinate activities of staff within another discipline — that is the duty of the responsible manager); [he will] monitor the services provided in the sector and participate in planning affecting it.'[43] This categorically prevents the administrator from intervening in the management of a department in order to achieve a goal which, in turn, affects the goals of the organisation. Monitoring rights appear small compensation and since, as has been noted earlier, the most senior managers are finding that concept difficult to apply, it is not surprising if this difficulty is being compounded at local level.

While there is no provision in the management structure for a sector tier as such, this 'fails to distinguish between the location of official authority within the District as a whole, i.e. the DMT, and the existence of several levels of authority, within the organisational structure of any one discipline.'[44]

One considered attempt to attack this crucial problem of local management has been reported by Spencer.[45] He has drawn attention to the arrangements developed for sector management teams (SMTs) in the single-district Oxfordshire Area, and these arrangements reflect trends elsewhere. He noted that the sector notion was 'somewhat shadowy' in the 'Management Arrangements',[46] whereas in Oxfordshire the SMTs are like 'mini DMTs', apart from a slightly wider membership, having some budgetary authority but responsible to their parent Area Management Team (AMT) rather than to the Authority and thereby also espousing the line relationship lacking in multi-district areas. The problem of reconciling functional budgeting by area officers with the role of the Oxfordshire SMTs (essential if the teams are to have a meaningful role) is resolved by:

> A mixed budgetary system [which] allows ultimate control to lie
> with the responsible chief officer but provides for a substantial
> degree of delegation of spending power to line subordinates who are,
> of course, responsive to pressures from their local SMT.[47]

Given the complexity of these relationships — notions of ultimate
control, a substantial degree of delegation and line subordinates
responsive to pressures — they clearly warrant rigorous probing
to establish their real operational meaning and indeed the whole
SMT-AMT apparatus needs monitoring (in the plain language sense) over
an extended period, before it can be judged to have solved the problems
of organisational relationships. None the less, the idea of continuing the
multi-disciplinary management team approach at sector level should be
judged a sensible one, but the difficulty is that the sector team, unlike a
District Management Team or Area Management Team or Area Team of
Officers, has no legitimised status and, unless the members which com-
prise it are particularly forceful personalities with the requisite political
influence in the Area/District organisation, then it is easy for it to be
side-stepped.

But whatever its practical merits or demerits, the Oxfordshire
approach is interesting in that it identifies the interdependence of senior
administrators operating in the political arena and the institutional
administrators ensuring the provision of services. But before proceeding
to explore relations between the two sets of administrators, the position
of the institutional administrator should be summarised.

Two possibilities exist for him at local level: a management role
implying control over the use of all resources, or a monitoring and co-
ordinating role of others with no control over resources. The
management role once accorded the hospital secretary or unit administrator has been eroded by the development of functional management.
This has made successful local organisation more difficult and the
management arrangements accompanying NHS reorganisation have only
exacerbated an existing situation. The weakening of the role of the
institutional administrator and the signs of his low morale indicate the
critical need for a reappraisal of the approach to local organisation.

Bridging the Management Gap

The inference from what has been said so far is that there is an evident
support gap between the 'political' tier of management (Area and

District) and the institutional tier (sector and unit); a gap that must in some way be made good. As an analysis of the organisational problems of the Health Service, this contrasts sharply with the vogue to bemoan the growth of the state bureaucracy by both press and politicians alike, in consequence of which the National Health Service soon became a ready target for attack on its administrative costs. But the hullabaloo about administrative costs can now be seen to be in fact a red herring—a means of acknowledging that there is something wrong with the new management structure of the Service without actually having to identify the problems. Red tape and over-administration are predictable criticisms of the public sector which will always attract an audience but are unconvincing as arguments, when costs and numbers are analysed in detail, and above all give no indication of the extent of the problems for the administrators who are struggling with a new and complicated machinery, and the consequences of the management gap.

There is in fact a more reasonable and plausible explanation for the administrative difficulties experienced since reorganisation. During the reorganisation of the National Health Service the provision of extremely generous terms for early retirement together with the introduction of what many regard as being an additional tier of administration had three important results. First, the Service lost many staff in the higher age groups who had held senior posts and whose depth of administrative experience was lost to the new organisation. Second, young and inexperienced administrators were able to gain appointments to many of the vacant institutional management posts. In hospitals lack of years has traditionally been identified with the right to take decisions on only the most minor issues and as a result decision-seekers now direct their attention upwards, regardless of whether the young administrator is in fact empowered to take positive action. Third, where posts were not filled by young administrators, they were often obtained by those who may have been unable to secure more dramatic promotion. This is not universally the case, since some officers have an entirely laudable preference for institutional posts and have resisted the pressure to move. But, it is true to say that the majority of experienced high-calibre administrators have not been able to resist the pull of salary differential which has forced them to seek posts as members of management teams or heads of divisions.

The widening gap between the two arenas of administration is most interestingly highlighted by the comments on unit administration of the Trent Regional Team of Officers in a report prepared by them on the management arrangements in the Sheffield Area. The Trent team noted

the critical judgement passed by the hospitals' professional staffs that
the effectiveness of unit administration had declined because of the
interposition of the Sector Administrator between hospital and district
headquarters. They concluded that the evidence they had received threw
great doubt on the position of the Sector Administrator:

> Hospitals appear to have been associated with other hospitals
> purely to provide an appropriate salary grading for a Sector Adminis-
> trator, irrespective of the functional relationship of the hospitals
> concerned. . . Other displines are not so organised on a sector basis
> and some absurd situations were described to us which illustrated the
> confusion and delays to which these arrangements seem to contri-
> bute.[48]

In fact their findings are, to say the least, debatable and their analysis
cannot go unchallenged. Institutional administration is weak because
sector status is also weak. It has no back-up support from above and, as
has been argued already, it relies for its administrators largely on the
young, inexperienced and less able. It is not surprising that in the reorganised Service, sector and unit administration are giving most cause
for concern.

Yet this problem is not really a recent phenomenon. As early as 1957
Noel Hall[49] made it clear that if hospital secretaries were not given suitable remuneration and satisfactory acknowledgement of status, then
many would seek too early promotion to group or region and *hospital*
administration would be weakened as a result. But the situation can be
corrected. Proper consideration of the respective responsibilities of team
administrators (and their immediate support staff) with institutional
managers would sensibly result in a narrowing of salary differentials. This
would bring long-run improvement in local administration and its feasibility is demonstrated by the way in which the differential was largely
removed in respect of Area and District Administrator remuneration.
As the provision of services to the public is the very *raison d' être* of the
NHS, the sector or unit post must be seen as a pivotal position where
decisions can be quickly taken and resources thus allocated for the services to be provided. It cannot be left as a post which embodies
inexperience and weakness. In these circumstances it is the responsibility of District and Area Administrators, and no more than common
sense demands, to establish the pivot. This would mean ensuring that
access to functional professional heads and administrators at the next
tier up is obtained only through the appropriate local administrator.

Similarly they can establish the pivot by ensuring that professional heads, at whatever tier, approach the locally based staff in their own discipline through the local administrator, rather than directly managing them.

A vital sector tier is self-evidently needed if the reorganisation objective of integration of hospital and community services is to be achieved. If administration at sector and unit level is not as strong as it should be for that purpose, that should not be taken as the occasion for other tiers of management to step in and take over the sector role. Instead, it is their task to establish the pivot and then to close the support gap to ensure that the local administrator functions effectively. If this is done then it is possible for both the 'political' and institutional administrative tiers to operate complementarily and successfully. Running the show from the centre of stepping in once the crisis has occurred, like some *deus ex machina,* is likely to be resented by local administrators much more than would no contact at all. The 'political' administrators need to keep themselves well informed of what is happening in their hospital constituencies, and they can achieve this by supporting their institutional managers: support of this nature is simply sound preventive practice. The District and Area administrators cannot afford to be constantly diverting their attention to local issues, but their own policy and strategic tasks can only be accomplished with the sure knowledge that the sectors are operating efficiently and providing a constant source of ideas and innovation.

One clear implication of all this is that the weight of administrative numbers must be at sector and unit level. It would be curiously contradictory if team administrators accepted the need to establish a pivot and to support rather than interfere, if the administrators at the 'political' level seriously outnumber the local administrators. This is a straightforward argument about chiefs and indians, and the resentment at a continuing imbalance of numbers is more likely to provoke local administrators to abdicate their responsibilities than to establish the sector as the pivot of the structure.

So the issues are resolved into one proposition; if the senior administrators are to adjust to their new 'political' arena and to master their ongoing tasks of policy-making and strategy, they must first secure the base of institutional management. They must look much more urgently and carefully, not at how they can *control* their sector and unit managers, but how they can *support* them. They need to demonstrate that they recognise an interdependence—one group with the other. Only then will they be able to claim a matching response from their institutional colleagues.

Notes

1. In particular see R. T. Golembiewski, *Organising Men and Power: patterns of behaviour and line-staff models,* Rand McNally, Chicago, 1967; and T. D. Hunter, 'Arena or amoeba: managing the health care network', *The Hospital,* April 1971.
2. A. F. Bradbeer, *Internal Administration of Hospitals,* Central Health Services Council, HMSO, 1954.
3. N. Hall, *Report on the Grading Structure of Administrative and Clerical Staff in the Hospital Service,* HMSO, 1957.
4. A. F. Bradbeer, op. cit., 1954.
5. W. M. Farquharson-Lang, *Administrative Practice of Hospital Boards in Scotland,* Scottish Health Service Council, HMSO, 1966.
6. *Management Arrangements for the Reorganised National Health Service,* HMSO, 1972.
7. *National Health Service Reorganisation Consultative Document,* Department of Health and Social Security, May 1971.
8. See C. J. Ham, this volume.
9. Association of Chief Administrators of Health Authorities (ACAHA), *A Review of the Management of the Reorganised NHS 1975 undertaken by a Working Party of the ACAHA,* December 1975.
10. HM(61)59, *Public Bodies (Admission to Meetings) Act 1960,* Ministry of Health, 1961; and NHS Reorganisation Circular HRC(73)22, *Membership and Procedure of Regional and Area Health Authorities,* DHSS, 1973.
11. HM(70)17, *National Health Service Hospital Advisory Service,* DHSS, 1970; and HC(76)21, *Health Services Development, The Health Advisory Service,* DHSS, 1976.
12. HM(73)52, *Health Service Commissioner,* DHSS, 1973; and HSC(IS)10, *Health Service Commissioner,* DHSS, 1974.
13. M. Davies, *Report of the Committee on Hospital Complaints Procedure,* HMSO, 1973; and HM(76)107, *Health Services Management, Health Services Complaints Procedure,* DHSS, 1976.
14. Statutory Instrument No. 2217, *The National Health Service (Community Health Councils) Regulations 1973,* DHSS; and NHS Reorganisation Circular HRC(74)4, *Community Health Councils,* DHSS, 1974.
15. W. M. Farquharson-Lang, op. cit., 1966.
16. W. M. Farquharson-Lang, ibid., 1966.
17. Consultative Document, op. cit., 1971.
18. W. M. Farquharson-Lang, op. cit., 1966.
19. *Democracy in the National Health Service: Membership of Health Authorities,* HMSO, 1974.
20. Statutory Instrument No. 1099, *National Health Service England and Wales, National Health Service (Constitution of Area Health Authorities) Order 1975,* DHSS.
21. ACAHA, op. cit., 1975.
22. ACAHA, ibid., 1975.
23. See S. J. Dimmock, this volume.
24. Yet it should not be easily forgotten that the administrator was often 'latched on' and that it was only the senior officers who were quickly and efficiently dealt with. Services such as transport, supply, personnel, maintenance of grounds, medical records, etc., were taken on in respect of former local-government-owned premises by administrators holding hospital posts which had not, in theory, been changed as a result of reorganisation of the National Health Service.

25. Sector is used to denote a sub-district level of organisation and management, representing an institution or a group of institutions or a set of services. Unit refers to a single institution.

26. 'Management Arrangements', op. cit., 1972.

27. B. Salmon, *Report of the Committee on Senior Nursing Staff Structure,* HMSO, 1966; J. F. Hunt, 'Report of the Committee on Hospital Supplies. Organisation', issued under cover of HM(66)69, *Hospital Supplies Organisation,* DHSS, 1966; S. Zuckerman, *Report of the Committee on Hospital Scientific and Technical Services,* HMSO, 1968; N. Hall, *Report of the Working Party on the Hospital Pharmaceutical Service,* HMSO, 1970.

28. J. F. Hunt, 1966; and N. Hall, 1970, op. cit.

29. The non-implementation of the Area Linen Services Manager post appears to have been the most well-publicised discouragement of this trend, but equally appears to have been the only nation-wide discouragement.

30. A. F. Bradbeer, op. cit., 1954.

31. A. F. Bradbeer, ibid., 1954.

32. A. F. Bradbeer, ibid., 1954.

33. A. F. Bradbeer, ibid., 1954.

34. IHA, *The Administration of the Hospital Service,* Institute of Hospital Administrators, 1951.

35. IHSA, *et al., A Report on the Role of Unit and Sector Administrators in the National Health Service,* Report of a Joint Working Party formed by the Institute of Health Service Administrators, the Association of Chief Administrators of Health Authorities, the Association of Hospital Secretaries, and the Scottish Association of Sector and Unit Administrators—published by the Institute of Health Service Administrators, 1976. There is a marked change of emphasis, in this latest report, from that which was evident in the IHA report of 1951. However, the Institute states that: 'The Report is expected to provoke considerable controversy and while it does not necessarily represent the views of any of the organisations which set up the Working Party, they are all aware of the importance of the subject and anxious that it should be widely discussed.' In fact the four organisations represented on the Joint Working Party are to submit separately the report to the Deaprtment of Health and Social Security, the Scottish Home and Health Department, the Welsh Office and relevant staff side organisations.

36. A. F. Bradbeer, op. cit., 1954.

37. IHSA, *et al.,* op. cit., 1976.

38. IHSA *et al.,* ibid., 1976.

39. Management Arrangements, op. cit., 1972.

40. IHSA *et al.,* op. cit., 1976.

41. NHS Reorganisation Circular HRC(74)30, *Management Arrangements: Administrative Management Structures and Preparation of Substantive Schemes,* DHSS, 1974.

42. Management Arrangements, op. cit., 1972.

43. HRC(74)30, op. cit., 1974.

44. IHSA *et al.,* op. cit., 1976.

45. J. A. Spencer, 'Shaping Management in Oxfordshire', *Health and Social Service Journal,* 10 July 1976.

46. Management Arrangements, op. cit., 1972.

47. J. A. Spencer, op. cit., 1976.

48. 'Room for Saving?', *The Hospital and Health Services Review,* editorial, August 1976.

49. N. Hall, op. cit., 1957.

8 MAKING REORGANISATION WORK: CHALLENGES AND DILEMMAS IN THE DEVELOPMENT OF COMMUNITY MEDICINE

David Towell[1]

The reorganisation of the National Health Service in 1974 is one of several attempts in the recent history of public administration in Britain to bring about improvements in services through the mechanism of large-scale structural change. Typically this has involved massive upheavals for the staff involved and considerable administrative costs, but has been quickly followed by doubts about what has been achieved and speculation about the need for further radical changes. In the case of the Health Service, the first major study to be published after reorganisation[2] (that of the Humberside experience) seriously questions whether it had all been worthwhile, and in the Service generally there is already much discussion of how administrative costs can be reduced and which of the tiers in the new structure might best be made redundant.

Such judgements may well be rather premature, but they can be partly understood through considering the nature of this approach to organisational change. First, and reflecting the influence of traditional management theories concerned only with 'formal organisation', main emphasis is focused on the changes in structure which can be brought about relatively quickly by legislative and administrative fiat. Second, these changes are specified for all situations by a standard 'blueprint'. And third, the way this blueprint is to be implemented is interpreted centrally (even when the ostensible and declared objective is to introduce increased decentralisation).[3] In addition, it is usually assumed that the benefits of these changes in increasing the effectiveness and efficiency of services can be largely realised through the introduction of more sophisticated management techniques, of which corporate planning and programme budgeting have lately been most popular.

By implication, therefore, such administrative reorganisations may not devote adequate attention to the changes in attitudes and values also necessary for real changes in the services provided, nor allow sufficient local adaptation to variable conditions; and for both these reasons, fail to harness the full motivation of staff in implementing the new arrangements.[4] Equally, the preoccupation with management techniques may distract attention from the essentially political considerations which are likely to be involved in any real changes in the processes by which decisions are taken and new patterns of services developed.

Thus, in the case of NHS reorganisation, the basic objectives were to encourage the more rational, effective and integrated use of resources in providing improved health care for the people. This was to be achieved through changes in organisation structure, notably through unifying the administration of hitherto separate services, and in management processes relating particularly to planning, consultation and multidisciplinary team decision-making. Rather more implicit was the need for changes in what can be described as the culture of the Health Service—the perspectives on health care, inter-professional attitudes and values—intrinsic in any movement towards new emphases and initiatives in health care provision. Clearly these latter changes cannot readily be accomplished by central directive and would in any case need to be developed gradually over a much longer time-span than the administrative restructuring.

Also left less than fully stated were the changes in power relationships required in order to achieve any radical impact on the prevailing distribution of resources, both between different types of health provision and between different parts of the country. This understatement has partly reflected the technocratic bias in much thinking about these issues: the tendency to assume that better techniques of analysis and management would in themselves suffice to accomplish such changes.[5] In addition, the past history of the relationship between organised medicine and government in the evolution of the NHS perhaps suggests sufficient reason why reforms affecting medical interests might also be thought to require an indirect and gradual approach.[6]

Against this background, the substantial redefinition and expansion of the speciality of community medicine at the time of reorganisation can be regarded as of fundamental significance. It will be argued that this new speciality has been loaded with a major responsibility for engaging with the long-term problems in bringing about the changes to realise these basic objectives of reorganisation. The most widespread and innovative new role in this speciality is that of District Community Physician. The Health District is the basic operational unit of the re-organised Service and the Community Physician is therefore engaged at the front line in shaping the local pattern of services and examining their impact on consumers. By focusing on the challenges and dilemmas confronting District Community Physicians, it may well be possible to provide a microcosm of the issues involved more generally in making reorganisation work.

This essay begins by recalling the objectives of reorganisation and considering the tasks prescribed for community medicine in relation to these objectives. Particular attention is devoted to showing how the original specification for the role of District Community Physician was conceived as a critical influence at local level. A look at the background to the emergence of this new speciality then points to difficulties which could have been anticipated. An examination of the progress made to date further suggests that the ideal role has proved very hard to realise in practice, with a consequent growth in disillusion among community medicine specialists about what they are likely to achieve. It is too early to make definitive judgements on this situation and more detailed study will be desirable, but a review of these early experiences permits an initial analysis of what is happening in the speciality.

This appraisal in turn provides the basis for suggesting a fresh approach through which strategic aspects of the Community Physician role might be more fully realised. Following the model provided by reorganisation itself with its universal blueprints for the new Service, the typical response to difficulties has been the issue of further specifications by the central authorities. In contrast, it is argued instead that such general guidance should be balanced with greater emphasis to an approach which can be described as 'informed incrementalism'. The essence of this approach is the *acceptance* that there currently exists at local level in the Health Service diversity in the resources and skills available, and in the problems faced. Starting from the situation as it is experienced in different localities, it should be possible to work in an incremental way to enhance the effectiveness of what is being attempted locally, in the light of broad goals for Service development. While this approach does not aim to produce uniformity, it should help to ensure the most appropriate mobilisation of skills and resources, and thereby have rather wider relevance to the situation now confronting the NHS.

Reorganisation and the Challenge to Community Medicine

The basic objective of reorganisation, that of encouraging the better use of resources to provide improved health care, was seen by the architects of the new NHS structure as requiring that there should be a fully integrated Health Service in which every aspect of health care should be provided as far as possible locally and with due regard to the health needs of the community as a whole.[7]

Within these general requirements and having regard to the deficiencies identified in past services as giving rise to the need for radical change, reorganisation was intended to promote the following more specific objectives:

integration in the planning and provision of all personal health services (including health education, prevention, diagnosis, treatment and rehabilitation) with each other and with local government services (especially local authority social services and environmental health services);
a wider conception of health care in which more emphasis is given to the promotion of health and the prevention of illness, to care as well as cure, and to domiciliary and community services as well as hospitals;
more comprehensive and systematic planning of services for people in defined geographical areas in relation to the needs of the patient-groups (for example, the elderly, mentally ill) to be served, rather than the institutions through which care is provided;
more informed assessments of such needs and evaluation of the effectiveness of services provided, implying a more rational and critical approach to current resource use;
greater innovation, and more rapid implementation of improved approaches to health care to reduce the disparities between centres of good practice and elsewhere;
full participation of the health professions, particularly clinicians, in the management of the service while preserving clinical autonomy in the diagnosis and treatment of patients;
more uniform national standards of care and strategic direction combined with decentralisation to allow flexible adaptation to local circumstances in the way national strategy is applied;
greater sensitivity to the interests and views of the public in the communities served (subsequently given particular expression in the strengthening of Community Health Councils).

In anticipation of these aims, the Hunter working party,[8] set up in 1970 to define the scope of the work of medical administrators at Regional, Area and District levels of the reorganised service, effectively recommended the creation of a new speciality, that of Community Medicine. This speciality was to be concerned 'with the application of medicine to whole populations or to defined groups, and hence with the ascertainment of health needs and how professional services can best be organised to meet them'.[9]

The Hunter Report further emphasised the fundamental importance to the specialists in Community Medicine in their broadened
role at every level, of grasping the opportunities offered by reorganisation, suggesting that to a considerable extent success or failure
depended on their contribution. As summarised in the subsequent
Reorganisation White Paper,

> their concern will be with assessing the need for health
> services, evaluating the effectiveness of existing services, and
> planning the best use of health resources. Equally they will con-
> cern themselves with developing preventive health services, with
> the links between the Health and Local Authority personal social,
> public health and education services, and with providing the
> medical advice and help which Local Authorities will need for the
> administration of these and other services [noting particularly]
> the especially important responsibility which these specialists will
> have within the district management for promoting the functional
> integration of health care.[10]

As noted earlier, the District is the basic operational unit of the
reorganised Health Service. It is at this level where services are actually
delivered that all the hoped-for benefits of reorganisation will need to
be demonstrated. It is at this level, too, that the Hunter Report recommends the distinctive title of Community Physician for the specialist in Community Medicine, and emphasises the importance of high-
calibre and consultant status. An examination of the experiences of
District Community Physicians therefore provides a crucial test of the
emerging contribution of community medicine in the new Service.

This point is further emphasised by comparing the similarities
between the objectives of reorganisation which have been identified,
and the four main components of the District Community Physician
role, as envisaged in the 'Grey Book'[11] on management arrangements
in the reorganised NHS.

First, the Community Physician is one of six equal members of the
District Management Team (DMT): the team responsible, that is, for
managing and co-ordinating most operational services, and formulating
policies and plans for these services in relation to the community's
needs for health care. The Community Physician shares joint responsibility with other members of the DMT for Health Service management,
and is expected to strengthen generally the team's competence in

planning services, establishing health care priorities and allocating resources, playing a major part in the resolution of problems of choice.

Second, and in addition to this work, the Community Physician has particular responsibilities in relation to planning and health information. He is to co-ordinate the various multidisciplinary health care planning teams, contributing his epidemiological and other knowledge of local health circumstances and encouraging the integration of services, so as to ensure that sound proposals are prepared for the DMT. He is also to work closely with the District Medical Committee and its divisions in drawing up plans for medical services, representing a concern with the health of the community generally, and providing a link between clinicians and non-medical administrators. And he is to be particularly concerned with developing a more informed basis for continuously assessing the community's needs for health care and evaluating service effectiveness, including maintaining a health profile of the District and keeping under review the provision of services.

Third, in his capacity as a specialist in community medicine, the Community Physician is to act as consultant to his consultant and general practitioner colleagues, assisting them by providing information on needs and advice on the effectiveness of alternative approaches to care, and particularly seeking to stimulate further the process of integration at different levels between hospital and extra-hospital provision, and between health and local authority services.

Fourth, the Community Physician has responsibility for the co-ordination of preventive services (including control over the work of clinical medical officers in public health) and some functions in relation to the local authority, which in some Districts include acting as the 'proper officer' on environmental health matters, in which capacity he is accountable directly to the local authority.

It is evident from an examination of this specification that *inter alia* as manager, planner, co-ordinator, link-person, catalyst, monitor, evaluator, specialist adviser and proper officer, the Community Physician has gathered into his role much of the responsibility for trying to foster the longer-term changes which will be necessary to realise the intended benefits of the new administrative structure. At the same time it may be noted that this mixture of activities, although perhaps grouped together for expedient and historical reasons, do not necessarily relate closely together and may not all require the same level and type of expertise.

It is evident too that meeting this ideal specification would be highly demanding, and it would be unrealistic to suppose that such a role could be easily developed, even where the incumbents have extensive training in the required skills and enjoy considerable support. The Hunter Report anticipated the problem of overload on the Community Physician in a suggestion that two such specialists might be required at District level. Hunter also anticipated that the crucial factor in much of the Community Physician's work would be the extent of his ability to influence clinicians. The attempt to encourage good practices, foster integration, and evaluate the effectiveness of existing services would all require working closely with particular sets of clinicians. Equally sensitive would be the Community Physician's role in decisions about priorities and the achievement of a better balance of services in relation to an overall assessment of community needs, which would be likely to impinge on several sets of clinicians at once.

In response to the predictable anxieties this would raise among clinicians about their 'clinical autonomy', the Hunter Report went to some lengths to emphasise that this influence would be through persuasion based on the Community Physician's expertise as a specialist colleague. It was regarded as important therefore that community medicine should be established on a par with other consultant specialities, and that the new Community Physicians would be accorded high prestige by the clinicians with whom they would be working.

In the event, the widespread creation of these new specialist roles, together with the need to fill posts from the recruits available, has meant that while many of the doctors now in post have extensive experience in public health or in medical administrative roles, few had comprehensive training in the skills which this speciality would seem to require. There has also remained a substantial number of vacancies which seems likely to continue for some years to come.[12]

The Community Physician posts have mainly been filled by doctors formerly employed by local authorities as Medical Officer of Health or their deputies. There is evidence that this field of medicine has traditionally been regarded as of low status by clinicians, particularly by hospital consultants. Public health work is traditionally low among medical students' preferences in their choice of speciality and social or community medicine has been a neglected area of the medical school curriculum such that it is commonly believed that this field has not attracted the most able recruits. Notwithstanding the major contribution of public health doctors to improving the general standard of health over the past

century, Gill (1976)[13] has argued from an historical review of
the development of this field that its low status derives from the
fact that public health doctors, because of the nature of their
work, have not been able to share in the clinical autonomy of
other doctors. Further, they have had to relate in their work as much
to public attitudes and political opinion as to the views of colleagues
in other branches of medicine.

For all these reasons, the idea that the influence of the new
speciality on clinicians would derive from its prestige was from
the outset looking a less than auspicious prospect. As Wolman
(1976)[14] was commenting at the time, the Community Physician
had only very limited tools to carry out his job and was likely to
depend heavily on the voluntary support of clinicians and other
health providers if any substantial impact was to be made. It is
against this background that the development of community
medicine in practice can now be examined.

The Community Physician in Practice

The progress which has been made and the problems which are
being confronted can be appropriately considered within the
framework provided by the four main elements of the ideal specification for the District Community Physician's role identified
earlier. The considerable differences between experiences in different Districts, the fluid nature of current developments, and the desirability of more detailed study in this area, all mean that judgements
presented at this stage should be regarded as provisional. Nevertheless,
on the basis of a variety of observations and reports,[15] it is possible
to make an initial analysis of emerging practice.

The District Management Team

In the first year or more after reorganisation, Community Physicians,
like other staff, were largely preoccupied with maintaining existing
services and coping with the problems of transition, in many cases
carrying a heavy ongoing administrative load which left little scope
for new developments. Here extra difficulties were caused by the
economic crisis and staff militancy, as well as the way in which reorganisation itself was carried out (including the delays in guidance
on planning, which was then regarded to be the basis for so much
else) and the problems in staffing the new structure. There is a sense
then in which few immediate achievements from the presence of
these new specialists could be expected. However, some Community

Physicians anticipate the danger of continuing to be overwhelmed by day-to-day management matters, and being unable therefore to give adequate attention to the necessary analysis and forward-thinking. In a succinct study by one DCP of his own use of time, Murphy (1975)[16] reports that 30 per cent of his time was being spent in formal meetings, while only a 'miserable amount of time (0.5 per cent)' was devoted to epidemiology, despite his view that this is the most important part of the work.

As Murphy also notes, the work of the DMT itself is by far the greatest single time-user. Some of the administrative load on the DMT would be expected to arise to the extent that there was indeed increased delegation to Districts, although it is hard to find much evidence that the intended decentralisation in the NHS is yet being realised.[17] Equally, however, pressure on the DMT seems partly to reflect the very limited degree of delegation that is being achieved within many aspects of District management. For example, quite commonly it appears that DMTs have not succeeded in establishing appropriate management arrangements for large hospitals and have therefore no management body at hospital level to whom they could effectively delegate. Even further away is the emergence of lower management forums which cross-cut existing professional and institutional boundaries in order to focus on the operation (as distinct from the planning) of services for particular client groups. There is reason to suppose from experience elsewhere that this lack of delegation will itself prove to be a significant constraint on increasing the integration of services at local level.[18]

A related concern of some DMTs is to clarify the appropriate work of the District and Area tiers of management, and particularly to avoid a line relationship emerging either between the Area Team of Officers (ATO) and DMT, or between particular officers. Some Community Physicians have further problems in clarifying their relationships with particular Area specialists in community medicine (most commonly perhaps the specialists concerned with child health and local authority liaison). All these problems are complicated in some Areas by the past roles and relationships among those now filling the positions in the new structure.

Within the DMT there are differences in the extent to which a 'consensus team' mode of working has been developed, and also in how significant is the Community Physician's own influence in this team (where his relationship with the two clinical members may be of particular importance). Quite commonly it appears that Community

Physicians see themselves as carrying the main burden of trying to achieve the objectives of reorganisation at District level, without the support of either a large department (as with the hierarchical heads) or an important constituency (as with the clinical representatives) to enhance their influence, and indeed without having yet developed the information systems which might add weight to their arguments.

Planning

The preoccupation of DMTs with maintaining existing services on a day-to-day basis is also reflected in the attention so far given to planning activities—particularly, that is, to the processes of strategic policy choice intended to bring about the more effective use of resources in the provision of services better related to the needs of local communities.[19] Although in some Districts considerable effort has already been devoted to creating a strategic framework (relating to imbalances in existing resource use and priorities for development) to guide decisions, elsewhere the view has been taken that any long-term planning is irrelevant in the current situation of uncertainty. More generally, planning is still tending to be seen as mainly concerned with ordering priorities for the use of any extra resources made available. In the light of past failures[20] considerable resistance can be anticipated for any new efforts to rationalise existing resource use, and even more so, for plans involving the redistribution of resources between services: notwithstanding that the Consultative Document on Priorities[21] makes it clear that (in the government's view) the economic situation over the next few years must make this the main means by which the overall pattern of services can be improved.

These problems are reflected in the doubts of some Community Physicians about how far their DMT colleagues (and indeed staff more widely) are committed to the objective of developing a comprehensive service covering community provision as well as hospitals and the promotion of health as well as care for the sick, to meet the needs of a given population. It appears that some DMTs are still devoting most of their attention to hospital services, and in the case of teaching Districts, the needs of the local population are sometimes seen as in conflict with the other teaching hospital interests of medical education and research.

In the 'Grey Book', Health Care Planning Teams (HCPTs)—multi-professional groups of staff concerned with services to a particular client group—were envisaged as a key aspect of the new planning processes, teams in which the Community Physician was to have a central role. Often, however, the initial enthusiasm for this idea seems to have quickly given way to considerable doubts about both the functions of HCPTs and their likely usefulness. Different views exist among Community Physicians about whether HCPTs should participate in planning or be more consultative bodies; whether they should focus on limited special problems of the District or deal more widely with the needs of particular client groups; and whether they could or should become anything other than pressure groups for the 'Cinderella' services. In this situation, particularly where there is a lack of support staff for these activities, some Districts have seen it as practical so far only to establish one or two pilot HCPTs. In view both of the lack of experience in planning among staff and the weaknesses in management arrangements for particular services, not uncommonly it appears that such teams have become displaced away from planning on to more immediate issues of operational co-ordination. The conflicts inherent in the Community Physician's role may also have encouraged some DCPs to exercise a less than central influence on these processes. After two years of experiment here, the further central guidance to health authorities on 'Joint Care Planning',[22] with its emphasis on joint planning with local authorities at Area level and an associated (if rather implicit) redefinition of the functions of HCPTs as District Planning Teams, is generating further pressures for a reappraisal of the appropriate form for this kind of planning activity.

One must also observe that the District Medical Committees and their associated divisions play a significant part in policy-making and the planning of medical services, perhaps made even more significant in the absence of multi-professional planning teams. Again the Community Physician has been ascribed an important role in linking the work of the clinicians in these committees to District management, and some are able to use their influence in these bodies to encourage recognition of wider community interests, although not all feel that consultant colleagues take their contribution very seriously. Some are also anxious about how long clinicians will be prepared to play their full part in the new structures (and this applies also to the creation of HCPTs), given the time-consuming nature of the committee work and the long period required for the results of this work to be seen. There is concern too that the complexity of the new consultative machinery and the scope for delay this introduces will retard acceptance of the new structure by clinicians and encourage attempts to bypass these procedures.

Underlying all these aspects of the Community Physician's work is the further important factor that while better information and analysis of health care needs and service effectiveness are commonly seen as a basic requirement for more rational planning and decision-making, the technical difficulties of this requirement, compounded in many cases by a lack of skilled support staff, have meant that often they have so far made at best only limited progress in this area.

Taken together, these observations suggest the real difficulties which face Community Physicians in linking the *technical* analysis of policy problems with the *political* processes intrinsic to planning activity in a system characterised by a multiplicity of agencies and interests.

Specialist Influence

Many of these difficulties are equally relevant to the Community Physicians' efforts to mobilise their specialist influence. Through their participation in the DMT, Medical Committees and Planning Teams, and more widely in their contacts with all staff, Community Physicians are making some distinctive contributions as specialists in community medicine. As suggested earlier, however, they often seem to have only limited influence in many areas which are still dominated by more traditional hospital orientations, and many are doubtful about how far clinicians are yet accepting them in a consultant role. Nevertheless, some Community Physicians feel that they are having an influence in increasing awareness among staff of the world outside the hospital, and at least drawing attention to the need for more attention to measures designed to promote better health.

Some influence is also being exerted by Community Physicians in the crucial area of fostering greater integration in the services provided, for example, between consultants and general practitioners, and between health and social services. Again, however, the evidence from studies of the care of particular client groups suggests that there are considerable barriers both to increasing the integration between related services and improving collaboration between different agencies. Recent research on the care of the elderly,[23] for example, has indicated how while each party (the client's family, general practitioner, social worker, residential home and hospital) may share at some level a common goal and be dependent on each other's services, effective collaboration in the interests of the client can be handicapped. Explanations can be seen in the conflicts which arise from each party's efforts to conserve their own scarce resources, the differences of view as to each other's appropriate role, the problems of communication and co-ordination which arise from the different organisational patterns of general practice, hospital and social services, and the different geographical bases on which these respective services are usually provided.

Against this background, the current emphasis on joint care planning between health and local authorities, and the extra finance made available to encourage this, can reasonably be taken as evidence that the original concern with coterminous boundaries of these two authorities and the establishment of Joint Consultative Committees (from the members of these two authorities) has even at Area level fallen rather short of what was intended. In short, the task facing Community Physicians at District level is clearly both highly sensitive and problematic. There may often be no consultative forum (apart from Health Care Planning Teams) which links health and social services. There may also be a mismatch in the organisational and geographical basis of the two services at District level, and there may be little or no political support for an activity which frequently appears to be seen by both parties as involving further demands upon existing overstretched services.

At the same time, in relation to influence on their clinical colleagues, another difficulty for Community Physicians in mobilising their specialist role seems to reflect some ambiguities in the meaning given to the concept of 'community'. The Hunter Report made clear that in their designation of community medicine and Community Physician, 'community' embraces the whole population of a given area. More commonly in the Health Service, however, 'community' is used to refer to what is outside hospitals.[24] Community Physicians can readily come to be seen then as representing community in the latter sense, i.e. one of the parts of the Service, rather than in the former, i.e. an integrated view of the whole, particularly when the Community Physician's previous employment was with a local authority. These ambiguities may then reinforce the ambivalent response of clinicians to the new community medicine speciality, a response that could be anticipated from consideration of the previous status of public health as a branch of medicine.

Combining these observations, it can be noted how different aspects of the DCPs' role are likely to interact in shaping their influence. The Health Service at local level is clearly a complex organisational system in which administrative, professional and political processes all play a part. The Community Physician is expected to exercise managerial authority as a member of the DMT, professional authority by virtue of his specialism, and possibly also further influence deriving from his latent representation of what are perceived as community interests[25]

and his own charismatic qualities. In acting as a specialist, then, the
Community Physician may find his influence increased because of what
clinicians perceive as the significance of his views within the DMT, or,
alternatively, decreased, because the clinicians resent earlier decisions
taken by the DMT for which he is seen as responsible. He may also find
a conflict between his consultant role with a particular group of clinicians, his subsequent managerial role in the evaluation of proposals to
the DMT in which this group has an interest, and his own promotional
role (for example, in arguing for more resources for preventive
medicine) which may implicitly be in competition with these proposals.
In short, managing the different aspects of his role will pose considerable dilemmas for the Community Physician and make it difficult for
him to mobilise his full contribution in each of these areas.

Preventive and Environmental Health Work

The other components of the Community Physicians' work, their
co-ordination of preventive services and environmental health
activities may be rather less problematic, particularly for DCPs with
extensive public health experience with local authorities. In relation
to the prevention of disease, however, there is limited evidence as yet
that Community Physicians are having much success in increasing the
attention given to this area. Indeed, the transfer of local authority
responsibilities to the Health Service has left some ex-Medical Officers
of Health feeling that preventive services are likely to be undermined
through having to compete with curative services for funding. What is
more, the possibility that from within the Health Service, community
medicine will be able to play a significant part in the prevention of
iatrogenic disease ('the new diseases of medical progress') still seems to
be an issue for long-term speculation.[26]

In relation to environmental health work, those Community
Physicians with 'proper officer' responsibilities can be spending varying proportions of their time on these duties but with the immediate
and unscheduled demands of, for example, infectious disease control,
likely at the very least to prove disruptive of other activities. Balancing
this to some extent, however, is the familiarity this work provides with
aspects of the local environment, for example housing conditions,
which are also relevant to wider issues in health care on which the
Community Physician might seek to be influential.

An Overview

These observations on the several components of the Community
Physician's role serve to underline how even a fairly limited definition

of what is currently practical in this role can involve a heavy work-load. It seems evident that the difficulties of this work increase sharply to the extent that Community Physicians seek to take on a more strategic influence in encouraging the development of a more integrated, rationally planned and community-oriented local Health Service. While in the most favourable situations, there is already some evidence of progress in this direction, more commonly, however, the Community Physician still seems to be only a marginal influence in the administrative, professional and political processes which make up the complex organisational system through which patterns of health care are shaped and delivered.[27]

It is also evident that while many of the problems confronted are similar, there are quite marked differences in the ways these problems are being approached by Community Physicians. These differences are inevitably influenced by a number of aspects of the local situation, including the stances adopted by DMT colleagues, the staff assistance provided at District level, the specialist support at Area level, and the past roles and relationships of staff in the new positions, together with what Community Physicians bring to this role by virtue of their own backgrounds, skills and training. By way of illustration, some of these points can be clustered together to suggest in outline two contrasting role definitions. On the one hand, some Community Physicians (for example, some younger doctors with more recent specialist training in community medicine) seem to be taking up a leadership position at the centre of the District stage (possibly as Chairman of the DMT), and struggling to make an impact through embracing positively some of the main aspects of the new role envisaged in the Hunter Report. On the other hand, some Community Physicians (for example, some doctors with long experience as Medical Officers of Health) have continued some of their past work as proper officers and been more marginally involved in District management, showing some reluctance to tangle with the complexities of the NHS (possibly not being much welcomed by their clinical colleagues) and aiming more to adapt to what they find than take a leadership role in change.

These divergences have led some influential commentators[28] to take the view that Community Physicians are turning away from the development of the new speciality towards the easier options of continuing past practices, whether through a focus on public health work or a preoccupation with administration. More generally in 1976, there is evidence of considerable disillusionment within community medicine about what the new speciality is likely to achieve, and debate about

what the speciality is, what it should be doing,[29] and how adequate
the training arrangements are for the preparation of its new members.[30]
Not surprisingly, these doubts have also been reflected in external
criticisms, not least from clinicians, which seem often to focus on the
extent to which community medicine specialists are a further brand of
'administrators' (a designation given some support by the inclusion of
these posts with those of lay administrators in the government's freeze
on administrative costs).[31]

Two further points are of particular significance here. First, it is
pertinent to recall that from the outset, a key issue facing community
medicine was seen to be its ability to influence clinicians, while not
infringing 'clinical autonomy'. In practice, the boundary round the
individual clinician's autonomy is not easily drawn and may well be
open to dispute,[32] so that to the extent that Community Physicians
do seek to shape services and influence standards through their
responsibilities for planning, monitoring and evaluation, clinicians
may perceive them as challenging traditional areas of clinical control.
Second, as the economic situation has served to emphasise in acute
form, the essence of management in the Health Service is a concern
with decisions about priorities. The Hunter Report argued that the
Community Physician, through his specialist expertise and overall view
of community needs, would be 'qualified to play a major part . . . in
the resolution of problems of choice'. Hunter also stressed the importance of persuasion, but it is clear that whatever the success of
persuasion, management teams in the current climate are still having to
take decisions, in some cases about cutting services, which are not going
to be readily accepted by clinicians (and other powerful interests).[33]
Moreover, while expertise and information may ideally be an important part of the Community Physicians' contribution to such decisions,
it is plain that the resolution of problems of choice ultimately requires
political decisions based upon the exercise of values. To the extent
that community medicine strives to be influential in such processes,
its problematic nature and its potential for mobilising powerful critics
can be readily appreciated.

An Incremental Approach to Future Development

These observations underline both the importance of the Community
Physician's role to the future development of the Health Service at
District level and the considerable difficulties that are being faced.
They also provide a basis for beginning to identify ways in which
realistic further progress might be made towards realising this role.

In the current situation, with substantial variations in what is being achieved in different Districts, it seems that to argue for an ideal version of the Community Physician role which many of those in post see little prospect of attaining, or to provide guidance which is widely experienced as unrealistic, is only likely to add to a sense of disillusion among those trying to make a useful contribution at local level. Rather, the desirability of an alternative approach can be suggested; one which accepts that the diversity in the skills and experiences of Community Physicians, the resources available and other local circumstances in different Districts, will make for different patterns of role performance. What should be possible, however, is to start from the current situation and the needs of Community Physicians in post, and work in an incremental way to enhance their effectiveness, especially in strengthening the strategic aspects of their role.[34]

This 'bottom up' approach implies that different problems will be tackled in different situations according to local priorities and opportunities. On the basis of these observations, however, three important issues can be identified which are likely to require close attention.

First, there is the key problem of mobilising the Community Physician's role as a consultant (that is in advising his colleagues as a specialist) in such a way as to encourage the changes in culture which are intrinsic to new conceptions of health care, greater integration in services, and positive attitudes towards innovation. In addition to expertise in epidemiology and the organisational aspects of health care, this aspect of the Community Physician's role demands considerable skill in working across boundaries to foster integration, and to support multidisciplinary collaboration. Particular difficulties can arise here in articulating the different kinds of authority (professional and managerial) which provide the basis for the Community Physician's influence in different contexts, and managing the potential conflicts between the DCP's consultant, decision-making and promotional activities.

Second, there are the problems involved in the Community Physician's responsibilities for the co-ordination of planning and the development of information systems. These raise issues both of a technical nature about planning processes (for example how to use scarce analytic capacity in the most productive way) and also demand further role skills, notably in the 'reticulist' activity—linking together the 'right' people on the 'right' problems—needed to co-ordinate planning processes in the complex structure of health care.[35]

And third, there are the additional problems of remaining confident about the basis for the Community Physicians' exercise of authority in different contexts, and achieving an appropriate division of effort among the several components of this role in a situation of overload.

Faced with these problems, the incremental approach outlined here might profitably be applied by Community Physicians in developing their own roles, particularly where opportunities can be generated for DCPs to share more fully the benefits of their experiences with colleagues in other Districts. Clearly there are some similar problems being confronted in different Districts, so that with the differences between various situations and the tactics being adopted, a set of Districts taken together constitutes something of a natural experiment in Health Service roles and organisation. As is already occurring to a limited extent in some places, groups of Community Physicians may therefore be able to establish a protected forum in which to review their own activities, consider problems and alternative solutions, monitor experiments and provide mutual support in the implementation of new practices. In this way too, innovations achieved in one District might be disseminated and tested in other situations, and Community Physicians could gain valuable experience in acting as consultants to each other.[36]

In focusing on the Community Physician role, however, it needs to be emphasised that developments here could desirably form part of concerted attempts to make progress on a broad front if the objectives of reorganisation are to be pursued more vigorously. Among the significant factors emerging from this analysis, for example, are the extent to which the DMT achieves a team mode of working and appropriate delegation to other levels; the clarification of functions between Area Health Authority, Area Team of Officers and District Management Team; the successful collaboration of the representatives of hospital and non-hospital medicine in the District Medical Committee; the role taken by the Community Health Council in representing community interests; the effectiveness of the Joint Consultative Committee and Joint Care Planning Team in co-ordinating planning and stimulating integration between health and local authority services; and the establishment of planning processes and information services in the NHS. In this context, all these factors represent conditions which would facilitate the development of community medicine in the Health Service, or put differently, indicate the constraints on what community medicine specialists at Area and District can expect to achieve without such wider changes.

In conclusion, these observations have served to underline the very considerable difficulties that have preoccupied Health Service staff since reorganisation and the long way there is to go if the stated objectives of this major administrative upheaval are to be more fully realised. It has been suggested that because of the Community Physicians' potentially crucial influence at local level, their experiences provide something of a litmus test for trends in the National Health Service as a whole. While identifying the many constraints on Community Physicians, these explorations have also pointed to some opportunities there are for strengthening the strategic aspects of this role, particularly where the support of colleagues can be more fully mobilised. Such development is likely to involve Community Physicians in widening their conceptions of the Health Service as a complex social and political system, clarifying the different bases for their exercise of authority in this system, and acquiring relevant reticulist and other skills, as well as bringing to bear more fully the technical contribution of community medicine to tackling current problems. At the same time both Community Physicians and their Health Service colleagues may need to adopt rather more modest expectations of this new role than might have been created by its original specification. Such modesty need not prove inconsistent, however, with Community Physicians accepting the main challenge which remains—that of gradually playing a fuller part in encouraging the development at local level of a National Health Service which is truly more effective in meeting the health needs of the community and supporting people in the autonomous management of their own well-being.

Notes

1. I am indebted to the specialists in community medicine who contributed to the exploratory study on which this paper is based (some of whom also commented on an earlier draft), and to the Department of Health and Social Security which funded my work on this study as part of a larger 'Project to develop Processes of Self-Innovation in Health Care Systems'. I have also drawn on the suggestions of my former colleagues at the Tavistock Institute of Human Relations, particularly Eric Miller, Colin Wiseman and Michael Norris.

2. R. G. S. Brown, S. Griffin and S. C. Haywood, *New Bottles: Old Wine?*, University of Hull, Institute for Health Studies, 1975. For an informed overview of the NHS in this period, see also: Nuffield Provincial Hospitals Trust, *Ninth Report 1970-1975*, NPHT, London, 1975.

3. A similar account of the influence of organisation theory on public administration based on Swedish experience is provided by D. Ramström, 'The use of modern organisation theory as a tool for planning in business

and public administration' in *European Contributions to Organisation Theory*, G. Hofstede and M. S. Kassem, (eds.), Van Gorcum, Amsterdam, 1975.

4. An unusual example of an alternative approach to large-scale organisational change which took these points seriously is provided by the reorganisation of the Royal College of Nursing membership structure, the first stages of which are described by H. Bridger, G. Mars, E. Miller, S. Scott and D. Towell, *An Exploratory Study of the RCN Membership Structure*, Royal College of Nursing, London, 1973.

5. This bias has been most fully discussed by P. Draper and T. Smart, 'Social Science and Health Policy in the United Kingdom: Some Contributions of the Social Sciences to the Bureaucratisation of the National Health Service', *International Journal of Health Services*, 1974, 4 (3), pp 453-70. See also Lee's contribution to this volume for further analysis of the inevitable conflicts involved in simultaneously attempting to provide more equitable and efficient health care.

6. For example, Elston's contribution to this volume explores in more detail, past and current issues preoccupying the medical profession in its relationship to the state.

7. This analysis is based on the statements made in the Department of Health and Social Security White Paper, *National Health Service Reorganisation: England* (Cmnd. 5055), HMSO, London 1972, and DHSS, *Management Arrangements for the Reorganised National Health Service* ('Grey Book'), HMSO, London, 1972.

8. Department of Health and Social Security, *Report of the Working Party on Medical Administrators* (Chairman, R. B. Hunter), HMSO, London, 1972.

9. Op. cit., p.7.

10. Cmnd. 5055, pp. 34-5.

11. DHSS, *Management Arrangements for the Reorganised National Health Service*, op. cit.

12. A further analysis of manpower needs and the likely prospects is provided by P. J. Heath and W. H. Parry, 'Community Medicine: Has it a future?', *The Lancet*, 9 July 1976, pp. 82-3, who report that in September 1975 there were 119 vacancies in the new speciality (40 per cent in health care planning and information posts) with no early likelihood of making up this shortfall because of the heavy rate of retirements (31 per cent of those in post) to be expected over the next ten years. This largely reflects the age distribution of those staff appointed in 1974.

13. D. G. Gill, 'The Reorganisation of the National Health Service: Some Sociological Aspects with special reference to the role of the Community Physician' in M. Stacey (ed.), *The Sociology of the National Health Service*, Sociological Review Monograph No. 22, 1976.

14. D. M. Wolman, 'Quality Control and the Community Physician in England: An American Perspective', *International Journal of Health Services*, 6 (1), 1976, pp. 79-102.

15. These include detailed discussions with Community Physicans from a small cross-section of Districts, the published comments of others, for example, D. G. H. Patey, 'The District Community Physician in Practice', *Health Trends 7*, 1975, pp. 28-30, and F. W. Murphy, 'District Community Physician–Activity Analysis', *Public Health London*, 89, 1975, pp. 262-3, views expressed at conferences, for example, King Edward's Hospital Fund, *Area Management Teams in Single District Areas*, 1975, and Brunel Institute of Organisation and Social Studies, *Notes on Conference on the*

Organisation of Community Medicine, 1975, and the observations of colleagues, particularly those involved in studies of Health Service planning processes.

16. F. W. Murphy, op. cit.

17. See, for instance, the recently expressed views in the Regional Chairman's Enquiry into the working of the DHSS in relation to Regional Health Authorities, Report to the Secretary of State, May 1976.

18. In a different but related context, the Central Policy Review Staff, *A Joint Framework for Social Policy*, HMSO, London, 1975, have recently argued more generally the importance of both decentralisation and a co-ordinated policy framework in encouraging integrated development to meet local needs. This argument is well demonstrated in work on rural development by E. J. Miller, *Integrated Rural Development: A Mexican Experiment*, Tavistock Institute of Human Relations, 1975.

19. As described in Department of Health and Social Security Circular, *Development of Planning in the Reorganised National Health Service*, HRC, 73/8, 1973, the forward planning function is composed of 'the research, analytical, and considerative processes which result in strategic policy choices and long-term aims' and 'the programming processes which result in decisions to put into effect specific courses of action within a definite timescale as a means of achieving the long-term aims, and to allocate resources to them'.

20. See, for example, the historical study by K. Barnard and C. Ham, 'The Reallocation of Resources: Parallels with Past Experience', *The Lancet*, 26 June 1976.

21. Department of Health and Social Security, *Priorities for Health and Personal Social Services*, HMSO, London, 1976.

22. Department of Health and Social Security, *Joint Care Planning: Health and Local Authorities*, HC 76 (18), 1976.

23. T. Dartington and E. J. Miller, *Geriatric Hospital Care*, Tavistock Institute of Human Relations, London, 1975. Compare also, on mental handicap, M. Bayley, *Mental Handicap and Community Care*, Routledge and Kegan Paul, London, 1973, and for a valuable more general review of problems at the social work/medicine interface, see J. E. Tibbitt, *The Social Work/Medicine Interface: A Review of Research*, Social Work Services Group, Scottish Education Department, 1975.

24. The further complexities raised by the concept of community have been much discussed in the sociological literature. See, for example, R. Plant, *Community and Ideology*, Routledge and Kegan Paul, London, 1974, and J. Scherer, *Contemporary Community*, Tavistock, London, 1972.

25. It appears that Community Physicians might find support from CHCs but, in appealing to this constituency, they would run the risk of acquiring what other staff might well regard as an unwelcome ally, given the less than enthusiastic welcome which CHCs have been given in some Districts. The nature of CHC influence is explored more fully in Ham's contribution to this volume.

26. See, for example, the view on this point of E. M. Gruenberg, 'The Future of Community Medicine', *The Lancet*, 31 July 1976, p. 262, and the wider arguments of I. Illich, *Limits to Medicine*, Marion Boyars, London, 1976.

27. Even in the much smaller organisational system of a single hospital, research elsewhere (D. Towell and C. J. Harries, *Improving Patient Care: an action research study of change in a psychiatric hospital*, Nuffield Centre for Health Services Studies, Leeds, 1976) has shown that this is

likely to be a slow process. See also D. Towell and T. Dartington, 'Encouraging innovations in hospital care', *Journal of Advanced Nursing,* I, 1976, pp. 391-8.

28. Compare the views of J. S. Horner, Chairman of the Central Committee for Community Medicine, as reported in the *British Medical Journal,* 31 July 1976.

29. See reports on the Annual Conference of Community Medicine (13 July 1976), and note the decision to review the state of community medicine after Dr Horner (op. cit.) had told conference 'there would be no community medicine unless the CCCM took urgent steps to redefine the specialty and what it should do'. For other medical views, see the debate in the correspondence columns of the *British Medical Journal* from April through to July 1976.

30. At the time of reorganisation, a crash programme of 'Hunter' courses was organised for doctors taking up the new specialist roles in community medicine. The Faculty of Community Medicine has now introduced a membership examination of a more stringent kind and University Departments (through three geographical 'Consortia') are engaged in providing courses in preparation for these examinations. An account of these training arrangements is provided by R. M. Acheson, 'Basic and continuing education of Community Physicians', *Health Trends,* 7, 1975, pp. 53-7.

31. A comparable and fuller analysis of the problems facing Health Service administrators is provided in Sunderland's contribution to this volume.

32. Symptomatic of changing medical awareness on this issue is the *BMA News Review* Report, January 1976, that, 'As David Owen made clear . . . if every doctor is not prepared to take prime responsibility for the economic and cost effective implications of every action he takes, the layman or politician will do so, with consequent risk of clinical freedom.'

33. Increasingly important here is the organised strength of other health workers, as Dimmock's contribution to this volume shows in more detail.

34. In the longer term, further strengthening of the work of District Community Physicians may be derived from the gradual availability of staff who have benefited from the new and more extensive training now being established in community medicine, and from a greater involvement of University Departments of Community Medicine with issues facing Health Districts.

35. The nature of public planning processes and the need for the development of reticulist skills in such complex systems have been analysed in some detail by J. Friend, J. Power and C. Yewlett, *Public Planning: The Inter-Corporate Dimension,* Tavistock, London, 1974.

36. Proposals for a social science contribution to action research of this kind, and a more detailed statement of what this might involve, is provided by D. Towell and E. J. Miller, *Developing the Strategic Role of District Community Physician,* Tavistock Institute of Human Relations, London, 1975. A similar but earlier research project, where again a national 'blue print' for new management arrangements (the 'Salmon' Report) proved difficult to implement in practice, is described by M. Fenn, R. Mungovan and D. Towell, 'Developing the Role of the Unit Nursing Officer', *Nursing Times,* 71, 1975, pp. 262-4.

9 PLANNING, UNCERTAINTY AND JUDGEMENT: THE CASE OF POPULATION

Andrew F. Long

Population as a policy variable has recently come more sharply into public debate. In fact, in 1975 the total population of the United Kingdom fell by about 2,000[1] and, with recent declines in the overall birth rate, concern has been expressed at the implications of these population changes both for the growth of the economy and its sectors.[2] Concurrently, population as a factor in the utilisation and provision of health care has been assuming unprecedented attention within the NHS. Recent publications on resource allocation issues and on priorities in health care, and the advent of an NHS planning system have all highlighted its importance in the construction of policy. For example, the DHSS Working Party on Resource Allocation within the NHS in its interim report[3] recommended that population be accorded a more important role in the allocation of regional resources than it had in the past. Clearly, resources must in some way be allocated according to the population: the problem arises in deciding what population and what indicators of need or demand to use. The Working Party argued that resources should be allocated through the use of a new formula incorporating, for hospital care, population, related to patient flow and case-load, and in the case of community care population alone. In their report of September 1976, the case-load factor is to be dropped and a new factor reflecting relative mortality conditions inserted.[4] Secondly, the advent of the new NHS planning system also stresses the role of population. In the circular, 'The NHS Planning System: Planning Activity 1976/77', population is seen as the backcloth for planning, in the sense of 'population to be served'. Essential facts about the population—its age structure, morbidity and mortality patterns—are to be collated in 'District Information Profiles'.[5] Population is thus seen as the context for planning and the basis for the computation of numerous rates and indicators of health and utilisation. Finally, the Secretary of State's Consultative Document 'Priorities for Health and Personal Social Services in England'[6] partially bases the choice of priorities on expected future changes in population size and structure. Changes in demand as evidenced by the Office of Population Censuses and Surveys (OPCS) in their national population projections are used as a basis for arguments about future patterns of provision and resource allocation at a local level. In essence, services for the elderly are growth areas whilst maternity services will be cut back.

What is common in all of these three documents is that population and its forecasting are used as the basis for discussion and as the keystone to future developments at both national and local levels. Clearly, at a local level the population has been and will always be of paramount importance: it is the consumer of health care resources. More problematic for policy analysis is the availability of *information* on the population of interest. What information is there? What problems arise in its forecasting? Are the resultant forecasts not only accurate but also usable? What are the financial implications of such forecasts? And, if the forecasts have in the past been inaccurate, what are the implications for discussion about priorities and planning in general? Such questions revolving around the population and its forecasting only serve to raise another more general set of issues concerned with information available to the planner, its use and organisation.

It is to these questions surrounding the population factor, as a microcosm of the information and rational decision-making debate, that this paper is directed. The paper is in two parts. First of all, it is necessary to stand back from the everyday concerns of decision-making and planning to examine some of the technical issues involved in forecasting the population, the problems arising in its forecasting, and ways in which they can be overcome, in order to see how from a technical point of view the forecasts should be interpreted. The second part of the paper is concerned with the implications of this methodological discussion for planning at a local level and for the current debate about resource allocation and priorities. The intention is to guard against the belief that technical analysis is both possible, desirable and sufficient, by highlighting reservations about the nature of the art of forecasting and indicating constraints on the demographic input to health planning. Over and above the *technical* considerations for caution in interpreting forecasts, there is the overriding addition of a *judgemental* factor, i.e. the weight to be attached to the demographic argument at the local level where the role of values assumes paramount importance. Through this analysis of both the technical and judgemental factors involved in forecasting, attention is drawn to a hitherto neglected area of debate and policy.

1. Planning and Population Forecasting: Prediction or Foresight?

Population forecasts are renowned for their inaccuracy. Planners, on the other hand, prefer accuracy and certainty. They want one estimate of the future population level. For them a range or a number of estimates is too problematic given the other information inputs to the planning process, with similar problems of inaccuracy and uncertainty. But if health planners are to have one estimate of the future, what problems arise in presenting it? What assumptions are involved? And to what extent can the health planners rely on this estimate in formulating plans for the future development of services? In essence, this amounts to the following problem: is there sufficient knowledge of the population, its components and determinants, to enable its future course to be forecas ted with sufficient accuracy and certainty?

It is first necessary to clarify the terminology in use when speaking about the future and its estimation. The terms 'prediction', 'forecast' and 'projection' are used seemingly interchangeably. Do they mean the same thing? More importantly, are they used as if they mean the same thing?

The scientific meaning of 'prediction' is quite precise. Prediction refers to the use of knowledge or scientific laws to arrive at a future value or estimate for the variable under attention.[7] That is, a prediction is based on knowledge of the laws and processes affecting, say, population. However, the term 'forecast', while it is used by some as seemingly equivalent to a prediction, for example by Keyfitz and Glass,[8] it is used by others as a more general term, notably by Brass,[9] to include estimates which contain a subjective or intuitive element. 'Projection', like prediction, has a clear meaning. As Brass puts it, a projection is 'the calculation of the future population size and structure which results from fully defined assumptions about the course of the relevant measures', for example, a straightforward extrapolation of present trends into the relevant future. To summarise, the terms 'prediction' and 'projection' will be used in the following discussion with the above meanings: that is, a prediction involves the choice of one estimate and is based on knowledge; and a projection is the examination of the implications of fully defined assumptions.

The debate, however, is not simply one of clarifying terminology but arises from the use to which projections[10] are put and to the feasibility or otherwise of making predictions. N. Keyfitz, in his article entitled 'On Future Population', illustrates the problems of the user of population projections very clearly. What the planner wants is a prediction, not a projection, a statement of what will happen (an unconditional prediction), not what might happen if certain conditions are fulfilled (a conditional prediction). As he remarks: 'The bridge between the two points of view is in *the choice of assumptions.* Insofar as these are realistic the projection does indeed forecast what will happen.'[11] [My italics]

H. F. Dorn, in a classical article[12] on pitfalls in population projections, speaking of the situation in the 1940s, illustrates the dilemma in the following quotation from Thompson and Whelpton's preface to their projections for the American population:

> It is to be emphasised that they [the estimates] are not predictions of future population size...They are, strictly speaking, merely statements of what the size and the sex, colour and nativity composition of the population would be at specified future times if birth rates, death rates, and immigration were to follow certain specified trends.

and in his following comment:

> But most readers obviously assumed that these sentences were merely a polite bow to scientific caution... It seemed incredible that demographers were merely doing sums in arithmetic for self-entertainment; they must be serious and really believe that the projected population estimates were in fact reasonable forecasts or predictions of the future.

Three points are at issue here. Firstly, at a practical level, the distinction between a projection and a prediction is irrelevant. The former is used as if it were the latter. Secondly, what happens when a projection is taken as a prediction? Is it accurate or not? The answer to this question is simple: historically, the projections-cum-predictions were wrong, and if right, only fortuitously so. Errors were not inconsequential, either; for example, on the 1955-based population projection for the United Kingdom, the estimate for 1968 was 5.5 per cent below the actual figure of 55.8m, a deficit of 3.2m people—and it is easy to see why.[13] One should not forget here that accuracy and inaccuracy are relative. A 5 per cent error might be tolerable in one instance, in another too large. It all depends on whether any new information on the inaccuracy of the projection demands the alteration of a previous decision. Thirdly and most importantly, the question of the feasibility of making predictions is raised. If it is not feasible, should the choice of one alternative, one projection, as the prediction be left to the layman; and how should this choice be made, by reference to further evidence or one's own judgement or experience—that is, intuition or further data?

Apart from the uncertainty surrounding any estimates made of the future, imprecision arises from two sources; knowledge (about causes) and data. To forecast the population, knowledge and data on the components of growth—fertility, mortality, and migration—are necessary. Mortality, although little understood in terms of causes, is stable over time and thus of limited concern for imprecision. Fertility on the other hand, is varied over time, its social, economic, and psychological determinants unclear. A similar comment can be made for migration, though its course, at least at a national level, is more stable. Accordingly, imprecision in population forecasts is not surprising.

However, as W. Brass argues, one of the main failures of demographers has been in educating the consumers of population forecasts in their 'inherent imprecision'. The projections-cum-predictions are 'inherently' imprecise, he argues, because of the difficulty, so far experienced, in finding sufficiently stable relationships to extend into the future. The essence of prediction is repeatability. Without it, prediction becomes imprecise, if not.unfeasible. And so, the user is entitled to wonder whether his subjective or intuitive forecasts could do just as well. Exactly how one should judge the precision of a forecast is an interesting question. Obviously one measure is to compare the actual with the predicted, that is, an *ex post facto* evaluation, using different data. But this is not really a sensible procedure on its own. One also needs to compare the chosen prediction with the other possible alternatives. Here, then, there is a measure not only of the reliability of the projection method, but also of the choice mechanism of one rather than another alternative as the prediction. In other words, it is not enough to say that by using the 1958-based OPCS projection for the 1968 population of the UK the wrong decision was reached, but that by using a different projection as the prediction another and now more appropriate decision would have been made.

William Brass is a keen proponent of the feasibility and importance of making predictions. Demographers, he argues, are happy to accept responsibility for the formal processes of projection, but 'are not prepared to take the further step of specifying (however cautiously) *the plausibility of the assumptions*, and thus to change the projection into a prediction'.[14] [my italics] However, on what basis should they specify their plausibility? Brass continues,

> It is true...that the scientific basis for the exercise is insecure... On the other hand, most demographers, including myself, believe that their particular knowledge of population forces and processes can provide something better than a technology for calculating the outcome of more or less misinformed speculations.

Perhaps this really is the rub: do demographers know enough to make predictions, and given this knowledge do they have the right data available to them, sufficiently up-to-date and reliable? If they have, why is it that their 'predictions' have been inaccurate?[15] So the debate resolves to the question: who chooses a projection as *the* projection, and on what basis?

One school of thought argues that accurate projections cannot be made because of a lack of data and of knowledge, and that predictions can only be made fortuitously. For example, data on changing patterns of family formation through evidence on the spacing between births is unavailable on a routine basis.[17] Such data are of value in identifying, for example, whether the present decline in the birth rate is due to changes in the timing of births (postponement of births) or to changes in completed family size, or indeed both. But, more importantly, there is a lack of knowledge of the social and economic causes of fertility and marriage, which makes it so difficult to project and to predict into the future.[17]

On the other hand, given this lack of knowledge, some would see demographic prediction as working solely from demographic laws and processes. For this to work the population would have to be divided into subgroups for whom change over time is regular and persistent and, therefore, predictable. The problem is in detecting such homogeneous groups. For the fertility component a wide choice of possible classificatory variables exists, such as religion, occupation and mobility between areas and jobs, although at present the only variables used (by OPCS) are marriage and family size.[18] A lack of concern about social and economic causes of fertility is tempered by the necessity for such relationships to be consistent over time, to have a close association with the relevant component of the population, and itself to be predictable. In any case, given that the relevant knowledge is lacking, the only approach would be to use what knowledge one has about demographic interconnections to the best advantage.

The crucial question that remains is, who is to choose one alternative as the prediction, and on what basis? Should it be left to the user of the projection or should the expert choose one alternative and only present that one, with his reason? At this point it is useful to introduce one further concept, that of a 'prevision' or 'foresight'. For it helps to make explicit one of the essential differences between a prediction and a projection, that is, the role of *judgement*, and also to indicate how one or another alternative population figure can be chosen as the 'most likely'.

De Finetti[19] draws the distinction between prediction and prevision, and between the logic of the certain and the logic of the uncertain. He uses the term 'prediction' in the sense of a prophecy, picking out one alternative as *the* future. De Finetti continues by pointing out the illogic of prefacing such a certain statement with the phrase 'I think' or 'I feel'. In making a prediction, one is saying it is certain that in the year 2000 the population of the UK will be... In contrast, De Finetti puts forward the notion of a 'prevision': 'It does not assert—as a prediction does—something that might turn out to be true or false, by transforming (over-optimistically) the uncertainty into a claimed, but worthless, certainty. It acknowledges that what is uncertain is uncertain.' Instead,

> the various uncertain events are attributed to a greater or lesser degree of that new factor which is extralogical, subjective, and personal (mine, yours, his, anybody's), and which expresses these attitudes. In everyday language this is called *probability*... *Prevision* in the sense we give to the term and approve of... consists in considering, after careful reflection, all the possible alternatives, in order to distribute among them, in the way which will appear most appropriate, one's own expectations, one's own sensations of probability.[20]

Hence, a prediction is a statement of certainty, a prevision a statement of uncertainty. Arriving at a prevision involves assigning to all the possible future estimates a number expressing their plausibility. This assessment has to be carried out in relation to one's own judgement about the validity of the assumptions made, on the basis of local knowledge and experience. Accordingly, the concept of a prevision brings into the open the essential *subjective* feature of an assessment of the future. The concept of a prevision also guides the discussion about the choice of one alternative as the alternative. In the light of the inherent imprecision of population forecasts, the impossibility of making predictions, and the planner's desire for one estimate of the future, clearly a choice of one set of assumptions, one alternative has to be made. In so doing, one is not making a prediction; one is only specifying that these assumptions, this alternative look most plausible, i.e. a prevision. One alternative, rather than another, is chosen by reference to experience, local knowledge or the validity of the assumptions made. The arguments for and against each alternative are weighed up, at a particular point in time.[21]

The aim of this section of the paper has been to look behind the demographer's projections to see why they are necessarily inaccurate, to examine the demands of the user of population projections, and to explore the possibilities of meeting the user's requirements. It is easy to see why demographers rarely make predictions. Instead, refuge is sought in projecting one set of assumptions about future trends in births (for nationally, it is as if deaths and migration are held constant), not even sets of alternative assumptions, although official (OPCS) practice is changing.[22] Such a strategy of presenting projections can be partially justified; there is insufficient knowledge and data. However, the user of the projection has *no* choice but to accept the projection as the best estimate of the future, as a prediction. In a curious way everyone would be satisfied, were it not for the fact that the projections-cum-predictions are generally wrong! For the planner would prefer one estimate, would prefer certainty, yet knows that certainty about the future is nonsense.

However, given the imprecision resulting from problems of data and knowledge, to project one set of assumptions is a hazardous, methodologically unsound and misleading practice. Several alternatives based on differing but possible assumptions need to be presented. This only raises another set of problems, previously existing but able to be ignored—who chooses and how does one select an alternative as the most likely future? It was suggested that the end-result should be a prevision, the choice of one alternative as the most plausible, after an assessment of their relative plausibility according to criteria of one's own choosing. Such an approach underlines the *essential* role of judgement, of choice, and of uncertainty in the forecasting process, while leaving the planner with one estimate of the future.

The above debate about population forecasting applies equally to any area that involves looking at the future. One's interest may be in manpower planning, forecasting labour needs in the labour-intensive industry of health, or in forecasting the take-up of a new service. Three issues are common to any such forecasting situation: the user wants one estimate of the future and preferably a prediction; to make a prediction, knowledge and data are required; but, in general, such knowledge and data are lacking. One appears to be left with the essential uncertainty of the future, and the essential role of judgement in making practical use of a forecast.

II.   Interpretation and Judgement

So far, several methodological issues involved in making predictions have been discussed with particular relevance to population forecasting. In this case problems of data and knowledge are pre-eminent. Such a methodological discussion, assessing forecasts, their assumptions and bases, assists the planner and decision-maker by highlighting problems of interpretation and applicability. However the planner's interest lies in a more specific area, looking at the population with an eye to future utilisation, morbidity and mortality. It is to such a focus that this paper now turns, specifically to examine four crucial questions. First, what problems arise in predicting the population at a local level? Second, given these difficulties, what possible solutions are there? Third, where does this leave the planner whose interest in a population forecast lies in it being just one variable among many in his equation? This is; how should the planner interpret (population) forecasts? Finally, what wider implications does the discussion of forecasting and its associated problems have for such current health care issues as resource allocation, planning and the debate about priorities?

Problems of Local Population Predictions

The cause of imprecision in predicting the future population largely centres on the future level of the birth rate. In consequence, as the levels of births and associated rates has always fluctuated markedly, attempts to project (and predict) nationally the size of population have remained vulnerable. [23] For similar reasons, i.e. fluctuations in the level of births at a local level, local population projections have not turned out to be any more precise than their natural counterparts. An additional cause of imprecision, indeed highlighting the problems of predicting a local population, has been (and is) the factor of migration.

Nationally a net annual outflow of persons from the United Kingdom has been assumed for many years, an assumption amply justified by experience. Although nationally migration's actual significance as a factor of population growth is likely to be small when compared with the numbers of births and deaths, locally this cannot be assumed to be the case. Migration may be all-important and numerically significant. For example, the recent immigration of expelled Ugandan Asians, nationally of little numerical significance, resulted in increased concentrations of Asians in particular local communities. This raises two questions: what data are available on local migration?; and, what effect does migration have on population estimates?

Migration has two specific meanings: first, internal migration within a locality, for example, a change of residence from one part of a city to another; second, migration in and out of a locality, for example, from one city to another. In addition to these longer-term trends, one may be thinking of temporary, even daily, migration in relation to place of work, residence, or holiday. For example, if one has an accident at work or on holiday, where 'should' one go for treatment? The repercussions for the utilisation, access and planning of health services at a local level are readily apparent.

The main problem of migration as far as population estimates are concerned is one of data. Using the example of mobility of residence,[24] there are three possibles sources: the census of population, the electoral register, and GPs' lists. The difficulty with the census is its infrequency and the prolonged delay in the publication of its findings. The actual data collected (on each person's address one and five years previous to the date of the census) are useful and complete, though there is no direct information on health. The electoral register is another source. However, its coverage—adults entitled to vote—ignores potential migrants (children) and it contains no other information except who lives where. As a guide to the simple numbers of adults involved in mobility of residence it appears to be a useful source,[25] but it says nothing about the ages of migrants, their dependents, or their health.[26] From a health perspective, another source might be the GPs' lists. But not everyone is registered with a GP, nor registered ncar his home, nor need or will a person register immediately upon moving. In addition, some form of record linkage of GP registers would be required to use this as a source for migration data.

Without this data, migration's impact on estimates of the future population size and structure is difficult, if not impossible, to foresee. The data which exist do not answer in sufficient detail the questions health planners pose, such as: what are the health characteristics of the migrants? What use will these new migrants make of the provided services? Will additional staff and facilities be required? As far as forecasting is concerned, migration is yet another cause of imprecision, adding uncertainty to that already created by future births.

It is also at a local level that the fundamental question of what population one is planning and providing health services for has to be posed and answered. There are two possibilities: a catchment population of, say, a health centre, a district general hospital, or a specialist burns unit; or, a particular population, collection of individuals, 'at risk' in some sense, for example, from a usage perspective (pregnant mothers, babies, the elderly), or from a social, environmental perspective (at risk of a coronary, of lung cancer). The answer to 'which population' depends on the task at hand. Sucha a conclusion is not closed to scrutiny. Adopting a slightly different perspective that health is about a person's 'complete well-being' (the WHO definition) that aim of health services is to promote and provide facilities for the treatment, care and cure of ill-healthy persons. The logical conclusion is to argue that one should provide and plan for persons *at risk*. In other words, one's focus should fall not on the child health population *per se*, but on children at risk, of being battered, of ill-health, of dying.

This statement leads on naturally to the question: how is one to identify persons at risk? Clearly again knowledge and data are necessary. What is required is first of all to isolate useful and usable 'risk' factors[27] and secondly, to identify individuals at risk, as opposed to looking at those demanding health care and cure. For example, two important demographic characteristics of coronary victims are age and sex; medical risk factors include blood pressure and cholestrol; social and behavioural factors include smoking, occupation and stress. With these seven factors one might be in a better position to predict a large percentage of the incidence of coronaries. But where to find information on the population in the health district specific to these factors is another matter. Information could be obtained from a sample survey on an *ad hoc* basis or use made of results from a national survey or one carried out in a 'similar' locality.[28] This raises a dichotomy in approach: on the one hand, to identify those at risk and intervening if appropriate; on the other hand, looking at those presenting for care/cure and treating, planning and providing appropriately. The former can be termed an active need-based approach, the latter a reactive demand-based approach.[29]

To summarise, problems in forecasting local populations clearly centre upon problems of data on, and knowledge of, the two key variables of births and migration. Once it is decided what population one is interested in planning services for, assumptions about births and migration must be made and forecasts computed. Again, one returns to the question: is one forecast based on a single set of assumptions a sensible procedure to pursue, or is the formulation and examination of several sets of assumptions and resultant forecasts and the selection of the most plausible by the planner, the better option? Uncertainty remains whichever way is followed, but choices have to be made.

The discussion so far can be restated as follows: population forecasts are innaccurate; such inaccuracy results from a lack of data and knowledge; perhaps the best that can be done is to examine the forecasts resulting from alternative assumptions about the elements of population growth to explore their implications for health planning, and finally to choose that forecast which looks most plausible, on the basis of experience. But does the user of a population forecast always have to cope with uncertainty from the forecast? Are there situations where the uncertainty disappears, that is, where one can make a prediction, or must one always make a prevision ?

Clearly, the answer to these questions is that the degree of uncertainty, the margin of error varies considerably, depending on one's focus of interest and on one's time horizon.[30] Births are the crucial cause for uncertainty both nationally and locally, but at a local level migration is an additional source. Accordingly, if one is projecting a 'population', for example the elderly in relation to formulating plans for geriatric services, where no assumption about future levels of births is required and where migration is minimal—in that the elderly in general do not move house, except as a result of slum clearance schemes—a prediction is possible. The uncertainty is largely removed. At the other extreme, one has the situation where both births and migration are involved—for example, a problem concerned with maternal and child services—and where uncertainty will likely be large. In order to minimise the degree of uncertainty—and thus the realm of speculation[31]—attempts could be made to draw up alternative estimates, based on differing approaches and sources, of the population of interest. For example, estimates could be produced of the total population of a district using the standard procedure (births, deaths and migration), or by using data on dwellings and occupancy rates, or by using projections of the number of jobs.[32] Comparison of the various estimates is then carried out and one selected as the prevision, the preferred alternative which looks most plausible.[33] In the event of each estimate leading to the same decision there is no problem. More generally, the necessity for judgement by the planner is still apparent.

The Interpretation of Forecasts

Throughout, the emphasis has been on the problems of making predictions and on the desire of a planner for a prediction. In contrast OPCS provides projections, in fact one projection and its incorporated assumptions,[34] although OPCS is now turning to what it terms 'variant projections' based on high, medium or low fertility assumptions. But what interpretation should the planner place on a population forecast? Unless the planner is willing to change his requirements of one estimate of the future, except in those instances where assumptions about births and migration are not involved, he will have to accept the inherent imprecision.[35] Certainty about the future is demonstrably impossible even to the wishful thinking in a situation of so little knowledge.

Other options do exist. The most satisfactory from a theoretical point of view is for the planner to accept ranges of population growth. However, as Thompson points out, 'if all inputs [to the planning process] have wide ranges, the resultant range of outputs is too wide to be of practical use in planning.'[36] Accordingly, all that remains is for the provider of the forecasts to spell out in detail the assumptions involved and comment on their significance. If the planner is made aware of the assumptions involved, he can modify them according to his judgement and his local knowledge. Being aware of the assumptions behind the forecasts puts the planner in a situation of knowledge instead of merely reacting to information.

This second option ties in again with a question raised in this paper as to who is to choose a projection as a prevision. Should it be the planner, with his local knowledge, or the provider of the projections? Some might like to argue that no one should choose; but this is to ignore the fact that choices have to be made. Given Glass and Keyfitz's comments that 'the weakness of population forecasts is due to our ignorance...',[37] it would be imprudent and impudent for the demographer as the provider of the forecast to pick out his prevision and present only that data. What is required is for the demographic expert to prepare a report indicating the assumptions made, the results, and his own choice, with reasons and preferably with a likelihood attached (resulting in a prevision). If the planner or decision-maker disagrees from his given state of information, or if his own evaluation of the consequences of a wrong choice demands, he is at liberty—especially as he bears responsibility for the decision or plan—to choose another alternative. As judgement is so clearly involved, it should be made explicit and reasons given for the choices that are made. Otherwise the basis for planning and decision-making becomes obscured in implicit yet essential subjectivity.

Population Forecasting and Health Care

In the light of the above discussion on the technical problems involved in forecasting the population, the interpretation the planner can place on a forecast, and the essential subjective component of any forecast, it is appropriate to examine a number of recent Health Service documents whose proposals are rooted largely in population data. Further, bearing in mind the problems involved in forecasting local as compared to national populations, it is proposed to consider the added complications in applying conclusions based on national data to local settings, where judgement and interpretation are the bread and butter of everyday working relations. The interim reports on 'Resource Allocation'[38] and the consultative document on 'Priorities' will be examined to illuminate and exemplarise the above discussion.

The interim report of the DHSS Working Party on Resource Allocation published in August 1975 proposed that population should be the crucial factor in determining the allocation of financial resources to regions. Four comments are in order in view of the previous discussion. Firstly, much play can be made of the question, what is the 'population' to be used for allocation? The Working Party make this quite clear: 'use should be made of mid-year estimates of home (resident in the Region) population for the year prior to that for which allocations are to be made.' In addition, where there are data on patient flows (interregional) these data are to be used in the favour of the region providing treatment. So, on the one hand, population data on those potentially at risk (in its broadest sense) are used; on the other, utilisation data (the source of the patient flow data) are to be incorporated. Secondly, this population base is to be weighted according to national expenditure patterns on the various aspects of provision—general hospital in-patients, out-patients, psychiatric patients. This serves to raise the question: why use national patterns of expenditure? Is the suggestion that national levels of demand and utilisation are relevant to local levels? Accordingly, should regions receiving additional finance spend it according to national expenditure patterns? It is only too easy to think of examples where this might be inapplicable: for example, areas with a large elderly population, or areas with a large holiday population. Thirdly, the population, especially when weighted, is used as an indicator of need. The Working Party point out its crudity as an indicator, and the necessity of

Table 2:   Changes in the Age Structure, 1973-2011, Great Britain (selected age groups: as a percentage of the 1973 figures)

Age Group	1973 (base year)	1981	1991	2001	2011
Under 15	100	89	95	99	95
60 and over (females)	100	105	106	103	108
65 and over (males)	100	105	106	103	108
75 and over	100	117	130	132	126
All ages	100	100	103	105	108

Note: Dotted line divides those born before and after mid-1973
Source: OPCS, *Population Projections, 1973-2013*, HMSO, 1974, Appendix
         Table 11, pp. 50-5.

further discussion and analysis to illuminate more sensitive measures, which are not unduly complex or cumbersome to handle and for which data are readily available. Given this comment, to incorporate a factor for patient flows into the allocation formula seems a little out of place. There is an addition of precision (utilisation data for patients residing outside the region) to an admitted crude indicator of need. If one's interest lies in creating equity between regions, why is there an apparent financial incentive to encourage favourable patient flows? In any case once patients' costs of time, travel and so on are taken into account patient flows become a disadvantageous policy. Finally, the use of population in the allocation of resources will demand the use of population forecasts. Without them, planning has no basis. Yet as has emerged, once a forecast is employed problems of precision and of judgement enter.

These comments have one common theme: what is the population of interest? Earlier it was suggested that an 'at risk' perspective should be adopted as a basis for the planning and provision of services.[39] However, there are problems of knowledge, on causes, and of data. Clearly, resource allocation is, and will be for some time, based on a crude indicator of need and demand, the population. Clearly an objective allocation—in the sense of everyone being in agreement—is not possible. As with population forecasts judgement and interpretation are the essential components.

An examination of the arguments presented in the Consultative Document 'Priorities for Health and Social Services in England' provides further and more extensive illustrations of the material discussed in this paper. Some of the population data used as an underpinning for the national policy on priorities are presented in Table 2. The figures for the elderly as a whole show a 5 per cent increase by the next decade, a stabilisation until sometime in the 1990s when there will be a small decline, and again an increase by 2011. Such variations in the elderly are caused by previous fluctuations in births, in deaths (for example, the influence of the war) and migration. For the 75-year-olds and over, a sharp increase is apparent, of 17 per cent by 1981, and of 30 per cent by 1991 and can be accounted for by changes in the level of deaths, i.e. increasing expectation of life. The picture for the under-15-year-olds is also fluctuating, an 11 per cent decrease by 1981 and then a gradual increase to 1973 levels by 2001. Here, the explanation is to be found in the variation in the level of births. It is apparently on the basis of such data that the Consultative Document proposes growth in services for the elderly and a cutback in real terms for maternity services.

The first point to note is the fact that the figures for the elderly are predictions: they will happen. This applies to the elderly as a whole and those aged 75 or more. Given the current usage of the health services by the elderly, as can for example be gleaned from reports of the General Household Survey, increased provision is required. On the other hand, the data for the under-15s are not predictions. They are projections, of what will happen if certain conditions are fulfilled. In so far as OPCS present only one set of projections based on 1973 figures one would perhaps be justified in viewing them as OPCS's most plausible projection for that year.

The plausibility of the projections for the under-15s can be examined by looking at its most crucial component, births. Changes in births and associated rates are notoriously difficult to 'previsage'. In order to look behind the data it is necessary to approach the future level of births from a broad perspective—women at risk, current family size intentions and actualities, and contraceptive practices. One of these variables only will be examined, that of women at risk of pregnancy. Until recently it appeared as though a parallelism existed between the trend in births and women at risk.[40] The reduction in the ratio of births to women at risk can only be the result of women postponing having children (or stopping altogether), of contraceptive usage becoming more efficient,[41] or of fewer women of these ages getting married or a possible mixture of these factors. Marriage certainly is not an explanation[42] but a tendency for a delay in child-bearing is apparent.[43] However, considering the plausibility of the projection, a large upturn in the numbers of women at risk is taking place with consequent implications for births, unless substantial changes in patterns of family formation are occurring—and here data are lacking. In other words, returning to the Consultative Document, savings in maternity services or indeed hoped-for savings in the education field may turn out to be nebulous.

The second point to note applies only to the development of maternity services: given that births are low at the moment and are not expected to rise to their previous high level at least for many years, can better use be made of current provision for maternity? In the Consultative Document an interesting picture is presented, showing a dramatic increase in cost (at constant prices) against a declining number of births and cases. Such a graph (Figure 5 in the Consultative Document), apparently quite clear, only serves to raise additional questions. First, what factors are included in 'expenditure'? An obstetrician cannot (overnight or in the longer term) become a geriatrician, say, or a midwife a mental health nurse. Second, supposing the data presented in the graph to be accurate, no comparison is offered as to the level of care provided in 1973 to that provided in 1970. No data are presented or even available, except in crude terms—deaths. In other words, the current quality of care could now be of sufficient standard whereas earlier it was not.[44] Whether or not the level of quality is both desirable and can be afforded is another, political and subjective, matter. In other words, can alternative use be made of current provision for maternity and, if so, are there any data to support objectively the contention that present services are running inefficiently? Without such data, the argument is one of values, not of evidence.

The third comment, and perhaps the most fundamental, is whether one can usefully argue from national data on local issues. As the document points out, local circumstances vary. Local levels of births, whilst generally lower than in the 1960s, may still be sufficiently large such that the quality of care is not as high as desired. Local changes in births will need to be kept closely under scrutiny, if any long-term redeployment of beds or staff is envisaged. The out-turn may present a fundamentally different picture.

The above comments on the debates about resource allocation and priorities underline two fundamental issues. First, if arguments and conclusions are based in any way on a forecast, problems of interpretation will arise. Unless a prediction is made, judgement has an important part to play in arriving at the forecast. Even then a judgement has to be made as to the weight to attach to the prediction in the formulation of policy. Second, the use of national data to support an argument to enlighten local debates is problematic, especially where local judgement and values are involved. Evidence is harder to refute. As both these documents employ population, its components and their forecasts almost as linchpins in their discussion, the role of judgement and values cannot be ignored, and so the debates must continue.

Concluding Remarks

The aim of this paper was threefold. First of all, factors involved in forecasting the population were explored in order to draw attention to the technical, demographic limitations of a forecast and thus to see the constraint on interpretations that can be drawn. Planners prefer predictions, but predictions require knowledge and data. These are not always available. In their place experience and intuition—i.e. judgement—have to be inserted. This raised the question of whose judgement, whose experience to use: that of the forecasting expert or the user of the forecast. This debate centres around the distance of the expert from the actual place of application of the forecasts and his distance from the planning and decision-making process. Secondly, some of the factors involved in forecasting the local population were examined. Problems of data and knowledge, of births and migration, were apparent. The fundamental question of what one's population of interest might be was also raised, resulting in the proposal that the desirable focus should be on those 'at risk'. Again, the role of judgement was emphasised. Finally, several current health services debates, which base their arguments to a marked extent on changes in population, were examined to see the extent to which the previous discussions illuminated their use of population and its forecast. Comments were made on the plausibility of the assumptions made in the forecasts, on the population of interest, on the role of evidence, and on the application of national data and conclusions to local situations.

Four general conclusions are apparent. First, predictions of the population are not possible. On the other hand, anyone can make a projection. What is required is the presentation of several projections, based on differing sets of assumptions, and examination made to discern the most plausible. If one can state its degree of plausibility, one ends up with a prevision. The demographer can legitimately choose one of the projections as most likely, but he should present all the possibilities, and the reasons for his preference, thus leaving the final decision on the most plausible projection to the planner. Second, the reason for this inability to make predictions lies in a lack of data and knowledge. More research on the causes of fertility and migration are required. Third, it is clearly problematic to apply conclusions based on national data to local situations. This is especially the case if some of the data are lacking and if some of the data result from forecasts. Judgement in both cases has to fill the gap. In other words, if there is insufficient evidence, objectivity, however defined, becomes an even more unlikely proposition.

The final conclusion and the common thread present throughout the discussion is the important, the essential, role judgement has to play in the interpretation of data and in forecasting. What data to collect, what assumptions to be made in the forecast—such questions have to be answered by reference to personal judgement, and the perspective required by the organisation needing the forecast. There is no other way to arrive at a plausible, let alone the most plausible, future. The uncertain remains uncertain; the task is to minimise its influence and gauge its extent. The result of this exercise is necessarily subjective, as it is based on judgement. Furthermore, it should be noted as being subjective and noted explicitly.

Notes

1. The population of England and Wales is still increasing, although births and deaths are approximately equal—due to net migration. See *Population Trends*, No. 3, Table 2, Spring 1976.
2. A recent collection of papers on the implications of population changes for social policy in general can be found in M. Buxton and E. Craven [eds.], *Demographic Change and Social Policy: The Uncertain Future*, Centre for Studies in Social Policy, London, September 1976.
3. DHSS, The First Interim Report of the Resource Allocation Working Party, *Allocations to Regions in 1976/77*, HMSO, August 1975.
4. DHSS, *Sharing Resources for Health in England: report of the Resource Allocation Working Party*, HMSO, September 1976.
5. DHSS, HC/76/30, May 1976, p. 24. Whether the preparation of information profiles containing relatively easily obtainable routine information (as opposed to *ad hoc* in-depth analyses of problem areas) is a useful basis for planning is questionable.
6. DHSS, *Priorities for Health and Personal Social Services in England*, HMSO, 1976.
7. For example, see W. Brass, 'On the Possibility of Population Prediction', 1972, p. 18, in C. Freeman, M. Jahoda and I. Miles [eds.], *Progress and Problems in Social Forecasting*, SSRC, 1972; or H. M. Blalock, *Social Statistics*, McGraw-Hill, 1970.
8. For example, N. Keyfitz, 'On Future Population', *Journal of the Statistical Association*, Vol. 67, No. 338, 1972; or D. V. Glass, 'Demographic Prediction', *Proceedings of the Royal Society of London*, Series B., Vol. 168, 1967, pp. 119-39.
9. For example, W. Brass, 'Perspectives in Population Prediction; illustrated by the statistics of England and Wales', *Journal of the Royal Statistical Society*, Series A., Vol. 137, pp. 532-70.
10. The actual methods of projection are also open to debate. See, for example, D. V. Glass, 1967, op. cit.; or E. J. Thompson, 'Population Projections for Metropolitan Areas', *Greater London Intelligence Quarterly*, No. 28, September 1974, pp. 5-10.
11. N. Keyfitz, op. cit., 1972. p. 347.
12. H. F. Dorn, 'Pitfalls in Population Forecasts and Projections', *Journal of the American Statistical Association*, Vol. 45, No. 251, 1950, pp. 312-13.
13. See OPCS, *Population Projections 1973-2003*, HMSO, 1974; also D. V. Glass, op. cit., 1967.
14. W. Brass, op. cit., 1974, p. 533.
15. One should note that OPCS indicate that the data they present are only projections. But the user almost has to use them as a prediction.
16. A deficiency which the 1971 census and subsequent censuses may remedy. Sample information is available: for example, M. Woolf, *Family Intentions*, HMSO, 1972; J. Peel and G. Carr, *Contraception and Family Design*, Churchill Livingston, Edinburgh, 1975; J. Peel, 'The Hull Family Survey', *Journal of Biosocial Science*, 1970, 1972.
17. D. V. Glass, 1967, op. cit., and D. V. Glass, 'The History of Population Forecasting', in C. Freeman *et al.*, op. cit., 1972, pp. 23-6.
18. W. Brass, op. cit., 1974, pp. 542-3 indicates the usefulness of these variables as discriminators for women married once only at ages 20-24 for the last 40 years.
19. B. de Finetti, *Theory of Probability: A Critical Introductory Treatment*, Vol. 1, Wiley, London, 1974. The earlier reference is to B. de Finetti (1937),

'Foresight: Its Logical Laws, Its Subjective Sources' in H. E. Kyburg and H. E. Smokler, *Studies in Subjective Probability,* Wiley, 1964.

20. B. de Finetti, op. cit., 1974, pp. 71-2.

21. The addition for the phrase 'at a particular point in time' indicates the essential time reference of a prevision. It is conditional on a given state of information. So one cannot be wise after the event: the information is different. N. Keyfitz, op. cit., 1972, and W. Fellner, *Probability and Profit*, Irwin, Homewood, Illinois, 1965, also utilise such a notion, emphasising the role of subjectivity and the importance of making it explicit.

22. For example, see OPCS, *Variant Population Projections,* HMSO, 1975. OPCS examine alternative growth assumptions, resulting in high, moderate and low population growth models. The models differ only in their assumption about the trend in births.

23. For example, see OPCS, *Population Projections 1971-2003,* HMSO, 1972; and for details about the basis of current projections, see OPCS op. cit., 1974, and N. Davis, *Population Trends*, No. 3, Spring 1976, pp. 14-17.

24. Information on other migratory movements is generally also problematic. But compare the data on journey to work patterns, for example from traffic surveys.

25. For example, P. Cross found a 98 per cent coverage of adults (when compared to 1971 Census data) in Hackney experiencing a net out migration of 2.7 per cent. P.Cross, 'Population Analysis in Hackney', *Greater London Intelligence Quarterly,* No. 30, 1975, pp. 38-9.

26. OPCS are in fact currently engaged in a study of the feasibility of extending information obtained in the electoral register, in the context of improving local population estimates. See *Population Trends*, No. 3, Spring 1976, following the report in OPCS Monitor PPI 76/1.

27. Useful and usable in the sense of: first, they discriminate between the various groups of people potentially at risk to a significant (both statistically and substantively) extent; and second, information is readily available upon these factors, or can easily be collected.

28. For example, the various reports of the General Household Survey (OPCS, HMSO) or such surveys as A. Harris, *The Handicapped and Impaired in Great Britain,* HMSO, 1973, indicate both the potential and the limitations of such an approach.

29. Compare D. T. Cross, 'Planning Forecasting', 1972, in C. Freeman *et al.*, op. cit., 1972, pp. 55-66.

30. The distinction in planning between the long and the short term can be contrasted with its meaning in demographic forecasting, between forecasts that involve assumptions about births and those that do not. In the former, uncertainty is large, in the latter smaller and so the plans or forecasts are less or more precise.

31. For births, information on family formation intentions and contraceptive practices could be examined. For recent studies see A. Cartwright, *How Many Children,* Routledge and Kegan Paul, London, 1976; M. Woolf and S. Pegden, *Families Five Years On,* HMSO, 1976; J. Peel and G. Carr, op. cit., 1975.

32. E. J. Thompson, op. cit., 1975, discusses these three methods indicating how they are carried out and the problems associated with them.

33. N. Keyfitz, op. cit., 1972, distinguishes five different forecasts and suggests that each should be computed, scanned, and that the user should pick his prediction and assess its likelihood — i.e. his prevision.

34. *Population Trends*, No. 5, Autumn 1976, contains an article indicating current (OPCS) methods of projecting local populations.

35. Compare H. E. Klarman, 'National Policies and Local Planning for Health Services', *Milbank Memorial Fund Quarterly,* Health and Society, Vol. 54, No. 4, 1975, pp. 1-28, and M. Buxton and E. Craven, 'The Policy Significance of Uncertain Demographic Change' in M. Buxton and E. Craven, op. cit., 1976.
36. E. J. Thompson, op. cit., 1975, p. 6.
37. N. Keyfitz, op. cit., 1972, p. 361.
38. At the time of writing, the latest report of the Working Party on Resource Allocation (September 1976) was not published. Its crucial component is the replacement of the case-load factor by mortality, 'to reflect morbidity', i.e. another fairly crude indicator of need. The effect on resource allocation to regions is major. However, the comments in the text still apply.
39. An alternative approach is to identify areas of deprivation. Compare the urban deprivation programme and the GLC education priority area scheme. See, for example, S. Holterman, 'Areas of Urban Deprivation in Great Britain: Analysis of 1971 Census Data', *Social Trends,* No. 6, 1975, pp. 33-47.
40. Compare N. H. W. Davis, 'Population Projections: the certainty of the uncertain future' in M. Buxton and E. Craven, op. cit., 1976. He also presents a population projection on the basis of very low fertility.
41. There is little evidence of this. For example, N. B. Ryder and C. F. Westoff, in *Reproduction in the United States 1965,* Princetown University Press, 1971, found a depressing picture with between 9 and 30 per cent of families planning both for the timing and number of children in the family. That is, the rest had at least one timing or number failure.
42. See D. Pearce, 'Births and Family Formation Patterns', *Population Trends,* No. 1, 1975, Table 2, p. 7.
43. D. Pearce, op. cit., 1975, Table 3. But ultimate family size does not appear to be affected (see Table 4).
44. For example, see the discussion in the *British Medical Journal,* 17 July 1976, p. 197.

10 PUBLIC EXPENDITURE, PLANNING AND LOCAL DEMOCRACY

Kenneth Lee

Ever since its inception nearly thirty years ago, the National Health Service has proved itself to be a continual source of copy for commentators. For some it has appeared to confirm the worst excesses of state medicine whereas, for others, it has appeared to offer a health care model capable of adaptation to other national settings; of one thing there is general agreement, it is big business. Indeed, according to latest figures, the NHS now consumes over 5.5 per cent of the GNP—the highest in its history—compared with the 3.5 per cent of some twenty years ago. Notwithstanding this growth in expenditure, accusations continue unabated that the Health Service is 'under-financed', the presenting symptom of the underlying conflicts and dilemmas that surround the political economy of the NHS.

In the first place, it can be confidently assumed that UK expenditure on health services cannot be insulated from the economic facts of life. The particular economic circumstances that the UK is now facing, and will continue to face for some years to come, necessarily heighten the debate about the role of the state in economic life. This in turn provokes the question as to what slice of the public expenditure cake appears 'appropriate' to devote to medical care, which may be reflecting essentially philosophical problems about the relative responsibilities of the individual and state. Although the health care dilemma[1]—that consumer demand and professionally defined need will always outstrip a nation's capacity to meet them—knows no political or administrative boundaries, the very act of 'rationing' becomes more evidently a matter of public debate within a centrally financed system such as exists in the UK. Government decisions to cut back total public expenditure—to provide economic elbow room for private industry—only serve to demonstrate more visibly that the economic management of the economy is a major determinant of the development of the NHS. An examination of the relationship between current macro-economic policy, public expenditure and present levels of expenditure on the NHS becomes, therefore, the introductory theme of this essay.

A second and directly related theme concerns the nature of the relationship of central government to health (and local) authorities. Whilst it might be expected that local plans and expenditure be 'consistent' with national economic and social policies, this tends to oversimplify the delicate nature of the degree of independence afforded to the subordinate agencies or periphery. By detailing some national initiatives, e.g. calls for standstills in public expenditure and proposals for revising revenue allocation formulas to health authorities, it is hoped to gauge more finely the reality of central involvement against the backcloth of expressed intentions towards devolution and local determination of policies.

Finally, attention is directed to a number of issues in health planning. Increasing pressures to control public expenditure in general, and expenditure on the health and personal services in particular have sharpened the quest for a form, or forms, of planning which would facilitate more effective and efficient responses to health care issues. April 1976 was thus conceived as an important date in the Health calendar, for it marked the formal introduction of a new NHS planning system. Although delayed by a period of two years after the reorganisation of the NHS itself, the Department of Health viewed the planning system as the bedrock of the reorganised Service. In the language of the Department circular, the planning system is seen as 'the main means by which priorities and strategies are evolved for the implementation of policies, leading to improved decision making and management of resources'.[2] Whether it will achieve the results expected of it can only be reasonably evaluated over a period of years rather than months.[3] Nevertheless, the essay attempts to track some of the important developments and issues in one potentially crucial area of planning — that of joint planning between health and coterminous local authorities — in order to assess the likely prospects for its acceptance.

Given the particular structural characteristics of the National Health Service and its emphases and initiatives in the fields of planning, priorities, financing and cost containment, this essay is addressed to such developments whether they apply at the macro- or micro- level. However, almost without exception, any prognoses offered are conditional upon a number of factors, not least that most roles and relationships affecting (1) macro-economic policy and expenditure on health; (ii) central policy and local initiatives; and (iii) the planning system and its outcomes, have yet to be worked out or are now in the process of being renegotiated.

Public Expenditure Plans and Controls

Any discussion and debate about the level of NHS expenditure cannot be divorced from its national context and, in particular, from the government's macro-planning and economic management role.

Events have shown only too clearly that the immediate key to projections in NHS expenditure lies in the immediate economic climate. As one senior Minister[4] expressed it—'the perennial problem of modern politics is [then] to contain aspirations within the bounds of the practicable'. Whilst economic growth continued, and the expansion in health and welfare provision remained unquestioned, it could reasonably be expected that NHS expenditure would rise absolutely in relation to national income. And so it happened, but the converse has yet to be tested: namely whether, if national income falls in relative or absolute terms as happened in 1975, the accepted strategy is to cut back in real terms on health and welfare provision. However uncomfortable a position it appears, the UK debate has now consciously to shift to discussing and devising social priorities appropriate to a period of planning for change and retrenchment rather than change and growth. In terms of the 1976 White Paper on Public Expenditure to 1979–80,[5] there will be a virtual standstill in the planned expenditure on health and personal social services, though the plateau is necessarily at a higher level than in any period in the history of the NHS.[6]

Given that the success of ANY government is to be measured in terms of its ability to achieve what it intends, there is one issue of particular importance. This concerns the government's ability to control the global public sector expenditure of government departments, public corporations, local authorities, and the like; which in turn raises fundamental issues about the nature of the relationship between central and local government. Accusations[7] have been levied at the Treasury to suggest that public spending has been out of control, accusations which have, not unexpectedly, been denied by the Treasury. Others[8] take the view that fear of social policy expenditure being out of control has been exaggerated, in that an apparent mechanical failure in the control system could often be attributed to an explicit political decison or to changes in relative prices within the public sector.[9]

Notwithstanding these assertions and counter-assertions, and that cash limits already exist in the main public sector building programmes, since 1976/7 there are two particular mechanisms to tighten the public expenditure control system: first, close monitoring of cash expenditure through the year, and a more continuous control of calls on the contingency reserve; and second, the imposition of cash limits[10] applied to about three-quarters of central government voted expenditure (central government, local authority and nationalised industries) other than social security benefits. These cash limits are necessarily administrative ceilings and represent the maximum amount which the government proposes should be spent on the services during the present financial year. In this they make a significant departure from previous practice; hitherto public expenditure was virtually inflation-proof in as much as government retrospectively paid authorities an agreed amount to cover jumps in pay and other costs.

The extensive use of cash limits is a new development, and in the first year or so the arrangements are inevitably experimental. Two factors which do remain unresolved however, are those of coverage and flexibility. Firstly, government has had to admit that there are certain items of public expenditure which are virtually uncontrollable in the medium term and to which cash limits cannot readily be applied.[11] The second factor is that a cash limit is inevitably a crude control mechanism which, by its nature, is insensitive to change. The assumption of the government in holding to cash limits is that there will be no 'substantial' room for haggling and negotiation, and the White Paper on cash limits threw almost no light on this crucial question. Given that the major unknowns for all authorities are the magnitudes and relative incidence of price rises, these problems are compounded in the area of pay settlements where national agreements lie outside the boundaries of local agencies to control. Predicting the level and timing of pay settlements will inevitably be a hazardous business for Health Service treasurers, to be added to their problems about capital approval dates and scheduled starts. Circumstances such as these feed speculation on how long the government will hold firm.[12] Yet, despite such speculation, it seems realistic to assume that cash limits will hence-forth figure prominently as a permanent addition to the battery of instruments for planning and controlling expenditure.

The Experiences of Local Government

Since few doubt the enormity of the economic problems facing the country, local and health authorities may respond more readily to the White Paper proposals and, to the extent that they do, the central—local balance will have tilted perceptibly towards central government. Yet, it is no simple matter to say with any degree of certainty where decision-making ends and control starts. To understand the complexities of the central—local relationship, it is appropriate to consider the experiences of local government—given that for the next few years the government is likely to be more interested in controlling its expenditure than what the Layfield Committee[13] evidently wanted, a restructuring of it. The experience of local government is significant for two reasons. First, there are the attempts, exemplified by the statutory collaboration machinery for health and local authorities under the NHS Reorganisation Act, to bring the NHS and local government into a much closer relationship, if not eventually fusion. Second, there is an apparent desire among those working in the NHS for greater 'devolution', and for confining DHSS matters to what are self-evidently national concerns. In this context, therefore, the reality of local government finance and local government experience of devolution in practice do offer a ready (if rough) parallel for the NHS to the difficulties that might lie ahead.

The major features of local government finance in recent years have been first, the rapid growth in real expenditure and, second, significant changes in the relative importance of its three main sources of income. Local government finances its activities by means of governmental grants, local rates and miscellaneous income, i.e. charges. Governmental grants are estimated to account for 45 per cent of the total revenue income of local authorities for 1975/6.[14] Although this appears to conflict with fears expressed that local government is almost totally dependent on central funds, it is nevertheless the case that aggregate exchequer assistance has increased steadily to its present level of 67 per cent (1975/6) of relevant expenditure (i.e. net of income) compared with 51 per cent a decade previously. In other words, though local government does have alternative sources of income open to it, its expenditure has been increasingly met from general taxation rather than from local sources.[15] Is local autonomy therefore at stake, as the dependence of local authorities upon central finance accelerates?

Historically, the purpose of government grants has been to reimburse local authorities for that part of their expenditure that was required to meet national rather than local purposes. As Layfield notes, its importance today lies in three other directions. First, that government has through its rate support grant attempted to redress differences in revenue-raising capability as between local authorities by resorting to a formula which includes, in ascending order of importance as sources of income, three broad elements—'domestic', 'resources' and 'needs'.[16] Yet Layfield was prepared to comment—'the calculations that determine the [grant] distribution may give the impression that the figures involved are wholly the result of an objective technical analysis; in fact they depend on significant subjective judgments.'[17]

Second, the grant is a block grant which means, in theory, that it comes as a lump sum with few indications (on the revenue side) to local authorities on how much they should spend on which services. The purpose of the grant can be construed as an attempt to widen the discretion which authorities can exercise and to respect the tradition whereby the final decision on local spending is left to the councils, who as elected bodies have a mandate to decide the services and amenities for their area. Again, Layfield feels bound to comment—'What has been clearly visible over recent years is a growing propensity for the government to determine, in increasing detail, the pace and direction in which local services should be developed, the resources which should be devoted to them and the priorities between them.' One might be tempted to summarise the position in terms of 'he who pays the piper calls the tune' yet, as the celebrated cases of Clay Cross and Tameside bear witness, the controls that may be exercised are often suspect, incomplete or exceedingly protracted in their execution.

Furthermore, given that evidence is sparse to support the view that uniformity of public service exists between and within local authorities,[18] it would appear simplistic to assume that local authorities are simply the passive responders to central direction. Although it is none the less true that local authorities are receiving increasingly detailed specifications of what the government would like to see in the way of 'desired' services,[19] it should not be automatically assumed that local authorities are little more than outposts of the central bureaucracy; or that local politicians, and indeed their officials, will allow this to happen. The conflict can be captured in this way: on the one hand there are public expectations for increasing standards of services, and the desire of those Ministers with responsibilities for services provided through local government to secure the execution of policies for improvement and expansion. On the other, there are political forces pressing for devolution and for increased public participation in local decision-making. Though this may be expressed as a polarisation between two possible sets, one relatively centralist and one relatively localist, there is in reality a continuum of choice about policies

The third main feature of government grants, and the one directly related to cash limits, is that rate support grants have been used increasingly as a means of regulating the level of local authority expenditure. Local government expenditure accounts for about a third of total public expenditure and as such is a key variable in the government's overall designs to manage the economy. Government's interest is not only in what it funds itself but equally in the amount of local authority expenditure funded from local taxation. i.e. the rates. Perceptible changes in the degree of central control can be observed in its recent call for a standstill in local authorities' current expenditure in real terms. Yet government has no direct way of ensuring those expenditure figures are realised and not exceeded. Apart from exhortations, and veiled threats about losing powers to Whitehall, the government's only real power is to reduce the level of the rate support grant in subsequent years. For what appear to be complex reasons, it is not possible for the government to operate this on a selective basis, so that resort to this method would be an extremely blunt instrument affecting all councils. But the issue cannot be seen simply in terms of controlling local authority spending. Rather, it is a matter of how far central government can go, ought to go and, indeed, is prepared to go in deciding national priorities and ensuring their implementation at the local level.

In practice, it may of course prove difficult to draw a clear distinction between the appearance and the reality of central control over local authority plans and expenditure, not only because of the existing constitutional and administrative arrangements, but also because it is often extremely difficult to monitor what services are actually delivering, and to what effect. But this is a problem affecting planning in general, and public expenditure plans for health and personal social services in particular; namely that no means have yet been devised to measure public expenditure plans in terms of the benefits produced rather than in terms of the money spent. With the rejection of the 'invisible hand' philosophy of applying the market mechanism in health, alternative mechanisms are needed for allocating and rationing resources to and within the NHS. Given that public expenditure plans shape and constrain the behaviour of the NHS, what signs are there at national and local levels that the picture regarding planning for health will be somewhat different or even better in the future?

A National Strategy for Health and Personal Social Services

One potential breakthrough was the publication in March 1976 of a government Consultative Document, 'Priorities for Health and Personal Social Services in England'.[20] One of the document's important functions, as the [then] Secretary of State saw it, was to provide detailed information to enable effective planning to be achieved. Justifiably, it argued that it did much more than this when it asserted that it embodied a major new approach to planning. To understand why this is undoubtedly the case it is necessary to retrace steps to a few years ago. Public expenditure on the NHS, although globally determined was, at the end of the day and with some important exceptions (e.g. approval fo for consultant appointments), broadly used to purchase resources in the fulfilment of priorities determined locally. Although this is in many ways too simple a view, a number of reasons can be advanced for holding it. On one front, many central policies and guidelines represented 'blue-sky'thinking in that they were policy aspirations rather than policy commitments. It may well have been the case that centrally there was no clear notion of what individual priorities might cost in resource terms, for no mechanism existed for costing policies. When the Department of Health advocated, for instance, improved services for the mentally ill, it was far from clear what money was necessary to implement the recommendations, whether that money was subsequently made available and used, still less was there much attempt to measure the effects. Furthermore, although capital works planning had always taken place in the NHS, particularly in relation to hospital developments, health services plans were almost exclusively related to the expenditure side of the budget. This policy satisfied the requirements of those concerned with financial control and audit, but it was less than helpful in describing either the activities of organisations or their outputs. Hence, there existed at national level a shortage of relevant information with which to analyse the resource implications of the policies being formulated and on which to base explicit choices between alternative policies.

Yet one might reasonably assume that a service publicly financed and run would be automatically subjected to an interactive centre-field planning system to determine the allocation of resources. Signs were indeed already appearing when, in 1971, programme budgeting was introduced into the DHSS with the main aim of relating expenditure to objectives. As with earlier US experience it was found difficult, if not impossible, in practice to structure health objectives and relate expenditure across to them. More modestly, therefore, a programme structure was established, structured in part in terms of 'target' and 'client' groups, e.g. the elderly, the mentally handicapped, and in part in terms of organisational frameworks, e.g. acute services and family practitioner services. For each programme an estimate of its current and retrospective expenditure was made, and, though in many cases these remain very provisional, they enable the main planning statements emanating from the Department to be costed in terms of annual public expenditure. Furthermore the trends of yesterday can become a basis for the extrapolations to tomorrow. The Programme Budget has in this way assumed importance as a major analytical contribution in the costing of policy, bringing cost estimates together to compare them with the overall constraints set out in the Public Expenditure White Paper, in order to determine centrally the broad framework of policies and priorities.

The need to establish within England a better national framework for determining national policy was only too self-evident and, consequently, the Consultative Document in its response to this need can be regarded as the first major breakthrough in national strategy, indeed the first systematic presentation of national guidelines in the history of the NHS. What is certainly new is that the NHS and personal social services were brought together with a clear indication of the financial resources likely to be available over the year 1976/7 to 1979/80, together with the government's views as to where its priorities lay. Yet, at the same time it is important to note that its conclusions and strategic thinking are by no means novel. Not for the first time has the emphasis been placed upon primary care (GPs, domiciliary services, preventive medicine) and the so-called Cinderella sector (geriatrics, the mentally ill and the handicapped). These have been declared priorities for some years but, as the statistics presented in the Document reveal, expenditure on the mentally ill and primary care became proportionately less over time and, even with the plans announced, the percentages spent in 1970/71 will be restored only by 1979/80, if then. The 'losers' are identified in the document as being the general and acute hospital services and maternity services, who will suffer a reduction in the proportion of the total NHS allocated to them.

Reactions have been mixed. Some regard it as a major political reform, an example of 'open' government; others add a heavy qualification as to whether it will really reform the present well-tried system of *ad hocery* in social planning. On a technical level it is difficult to predict how quickly and smoothly these policies could be implemented, for areas and districts will find it difficult to derive programme budgets on the DHSS model. Again, the constraints on public expenditure and policies of resource allocation will cause extreme difficulties within those authorities where cutbacks are much more than paper exercises but where staff redundancies are expected to be avoided. Furthermore, there is a genuine difficulty in translating general guidelines into local terms, exacerbated by a growing belief that the guidelines are in many instances unrealistic. Indeed in some of the fields of projected growth there would appear to be unacceptably large shortfalls between the levels of current provision and national guidelines as to deny the latter any credibility.[21] Finally, the implicit assumption underpinning most of the document—that switching resources from the acute sector to community care will in some ways reduce demands upon the former—is as yet unproven and may turn out to be as illusory as the original claims made of the NHS. Indeed, it may simply create new demands previously unmet or unrecognised.

Yet, whether these steps are too tentative or not in the right direction is, in a sense, peripheral to the central issue: the status of the document in the eyes of both central government and its local agents. There would appear to be little doubt that the primary objective is to influence the pattern of spending by peripheral authorities: 'It is on the balance of priority between these policies, rather than the policies themselves, that we are primarily inviting views' (page 5). Attention is again drawn to the paradox between the devolution of power promised under NHS reorganisation and this document, which some would strongly argue implies a form of central direction. If the agencies of local government and health are to be left *in practice* to choose how they distribute their funds then national priorities become no more than an exercise in rhetoric. If, on the other hand, central government is to determine priorities then local initiatives are at the very least circumscribed. The unknown in the equation remains: to what extent will local and health authorities be free to interpret in their own way the policy guidelines offered by the Department? and will planning teams be able to apply their own criteria on the adequacy of particular local services?

Operational Frameworks for Planning and Resource Allocation

The strategic guidance issued by the Department as a product of its own planning activity—the Consultative Document—is intended to form the strategic backcloth to NHS planning. Common purpose as between the centre and the localities is envisaged in terms of the DHSS planning system and NHS planning system interacting at the national strategic level each year. Although this is offered as the theoretical solution, the question is prompted whether, if centre and periphery are intended to interact in the manner suggested, either can afford to be seen to be the servant of the other?

One debate which neatly illuminates this dichotomy at the present time is that of resource allocation. Two major issues arise on resource allocation: the first concerns the proportion of national income that goes to the NHS; the second, the criteria by which available resources are shared out within the NHS. With the second, historically revenue and capital allocations have been made from DHSS to agencies representing hospital, community and family practitioner services without there ever having been a universally agreed set of criteria underpinning their allocation. For example, although the NHS might claim on some counts that it has removed the inequalities that a price system creates —ability to pay—it has allegedly failed to rectify geographical inequalities which are as serious. Although geographical imbalances in the distribution of medical resources—as judged largely by financial

yardsticks—is an international problem, sufficient evidence[22] existed of
its presence and scale within the UK for it to have become a matter of
public concern; the debate ranging widely over both the concepts and
methods by which NHS capital and revenue resources could more effectively and equitably be distributed through the country in response to
'relative health needs'.

Yet conflict only rises to the surface when the question is asked—
who will seek to change the existing state of distribution and what criteria and indicators are to be deployed in devising alternative methods
for allocating resources? Since the NHS is a significant redistributive
agent of both income and wealth, how far and in what direction this
should be carried out is ultimately a matter of political philosophy.
It may or may not come as a surprise, therefore, to observe that Ministers have been making the running, seeking more finely tuned methods
of determining resource allocation between different Regional health
authorities. Indeed, they have appeared anxious to devise ways of identifying Areas and Districts which are particularly deficient in health
care provision, with the prime objective of inviting health authorities
to reallocate their own resources accordingly.

The methods used to establish the formula for regional revenue dis-
tributions for hospital and community services for 1976/77 were the
outcome of a joint DHSS/NHS Working Party set up in May 1975. An
Interim Report[23] was produced in August 1975, the main features of
which were accepted and acted upon by the Secretary of State in determining revenue allocations to Regions in March 1976. The main revenue
determinants for 1976/7 were the population statistics weighted to reflect the use made nationally of different services by men and women of
different ages, and case-loads in hospitals. The recommendations contained in the final report now published[24] would, if implemented,
further refine the formula by dispensing with the case-load factors, and
by introducing a weighting of the population age/sex structure to both
the use made of hospital beds and mortality experience between different regions. The allocation of capital would also broadly depend upon
a basis of population weighting. As with the interim report, the final
version includes an invitation to regions to carry out similar reallocations
within their boundaries.

A number of observations can be made by way of commentary. The
first of these concerns the practical feasibility of adopting a Robin
Hood policy—of robbing the rich to help the poor—at a time when
economic pressures are causing AHAs to cut back in real terms. Equally,
doubts must remain as to whether the 'poor' can economically handle

the rate of expansion in human and capital resources assumed to be possible under the formula; it is not simply a question of a time-lag in building the hospitals but of whether extra staff can be recruited in such sizeable numbers. The second point is to question the desirability of the basic criterion selected which, essentially, is that each area should have the same value of resources at its disposal in relation to the population it serves. Whether this approach ignores wider epidemiological, social and environmental factors depends on whether the weighted population data used are reliable proxy indicators of 'need' or not. 'Territorial justice' based on *per capita* provision does implicitly assume that the health needs of an area are proportional to the size of its population and do not vary significantly with other factors, an assumption that will now be held up to closer scrutiny. For the situation is one of possible conflict between national notions of 'territorial justice' and locally perceived 'needs', the conflict only being minimised to the extent that their respective notions of 'need' can be reconciled. Cast in different clothes, they are the old issues—as yet unresolved—of how much we are one nation and one people...and who decides?

Further, apart from noting that there is a point at which the ideal of equalisation comes up against the ideal of devolved responsibility, there are grounds for doubting whether a policy of equality[25] in the distribution of 'inputs' would result in an efficient and effective delivery of health services nation-wide. Or stated more positively: the pursuit of an equitable distribution may be quite different in its effect from an allocation aimed at obtaining the greatest improvement of health. As Butler[26] points out in relation to general practice:

> Manpower planning which is based on an 'adequate' or 'equitable' level based in relation to doctor/patient ratios in other areas, is vulnerable to the charge of failing to discriminate between places with different patterns of social welfare provision, health care needs, access costs and so on.

In other words, whilst such ratios might be marginally useful as general guidelines for overall planning, they may not be sensitive or sophisticated enough to adjust for the relative needs of different population groups. In these terms optimisation on one front may frustrate optimisation of resources by another route.

Yet, in defence of this system, it might be concluded that the added complexity of moving towards a form of output or outcome planning is simply too challenging and costly at the present time, though the point remains that a policy based upon 'equality of inputs' takes no direct account of, for example, the cost-effectiveness of each area's performance. Many factors, including the spatial distribution of the population of the area and the legacy of buildings and equipment with which the Health Service in the area must function, affect the expenditure required to achieve a particular standard of service. But equally, wide variations in utilisation rates for specific diseases indicate that there is considerable uncertainty about the effectiveness of different levels of aggregrate, as well as specific kinds of health services.

Yet, paradoxically, a movement towards a more equal distribution of financial resources for health care may turn out to be counterproductive on the very grounds it is trying to achieve, namely of improving total social welfare. Confidence in a policy of equalising health resources between localities must rest on a belief that everything else in the 'galaxy' of human life is given, equal and constant between and within these localities. To relax these assumptions is to acknowledge that inequalities in health provision, when adopted as indicators of 'deprivation', cannot be separated from other interconnecting and cumulative forms of inequalities of class, income, housing and living standards — and even this might be too narrow for many people.[27] Given that material and environmental deficiences are more prevalent in some areas than in others, do these tie up with deprived regions and areas in health terms?—and, if not, should they?

To adopt that stance requires shifting our attention from inequalities on the distribution of health facilities to the nature of inequalities and deprivation in the areas. Two reasons stand out. In the first place, Townsend concludes (from as yet unpublished survey material) that an area strategy cannot be the cardinal means for dealing with underprivilege—

> However economically or socially deprived areas are defined, unless nearly half the areas in the country are included, there will be more poor persons or poor children living outside than within. With all or nearly all priority areas there will be more persons who are not deprived than there are deprived.[28]

Although this would appear to be an indictment of past policy initiatives aimed at, for example, urban aid and educational priority areas, it has lessons for the Health Service in attempting to focus solely upon area deprivation rather than patient deprivation.

In the second place, are we to conclude from the NHS resource reallocation exercise that government is more interested in geographical than in social differences to explain inequalities of access[29] to health care? Certainly there now appears to be growing evidence of clear social class gradients in the use of health facilities. Although these may be attributed in part to the operation of the inverse care law—the availability of good medical care tends to vary inversely with the need for it in the population served—Cartwright and O'Brien cite 'other mechanisms contributing to the unequal use and availability of health services [which] are all highly related—knowledge, education, attitudes, diffidence, self-confidence, vulnerability and the influence of these on the relationship between patients and doctors'.[30] It might be expected, therefore, that the measurement of deprivation will prove to be a complex task[31] but equally, we can at least conclude that the way forward is unlikely to lie in largely unco-ordinated attempts made by single agencies. What chance is there then for multi-agency approaches to social planning and multiple deprivation?

Joint Approaches to Planning

In terms of central initiatives towards joint planning, potentially the most important document to appear in recent times was published in 1975, entitled 'A Joint Framework for Social Policy' (JASP),[32] it emanated from a Cabinet think-tank—the Central Policy Review Staff—its aim being to promote work towards a coherent national policy for social planning. With some justification the document asserts that most social problems cross departmental boundaries which makes it difficult for any government to 'see and deal with people in the round'. Their indictment of the present way in which policies are formulated is levelled at the frequency with which policies, which should cross departmental boundaries in practice, are responded to by individual government Departments acting largely in isolation of each other. The JASP programme rests on two sets of proposals. One is to improve the way social decisions are taken, and to improve the information base to back them up. The other concerns investigations into specific policy areas which overlap departmental boundaries e.g. housing the elderly, social welfare programmes for the disabled. The document points out that if the structure of social expenditure is not to become increasingly arbitrary, some better basis is needed for defining national priorities and for formulating comprehensive strategies towards social policies.

Whether we are witnessing the birth of a new co-ordinated strategy for social policies—a movement towards national long-term planning—

is debatable for the following reasons. For its initial success JASP rests on the key assumption that if a 'joint' or more coherent approach to social planning is to have any chance of succeeding, Ministers and their Departments must be prepared to concede ground. Certainly, DHSS is regarded as being sympathetic to the philosophy but given its own jumbo creation in the late sixties perhaps it is easy for it to acknowledge the rationale; others may be less easily persuaded. One reason may not be too hard to find; Ministers and civil servants see their prime task, and in many cases their careers, in terms of promoting or defending the interests of the services they are responsible for and for asserting the independent capabilities of their departments.[33] Accordingly, it is argued, Whitehall departments tend to think departmentally and interdepartmental activity tends to be secondary. As Heclo and Wildavsky note:—

> Spending ministers do not acquire the name for nothing...Ministerial responsibility means that the department's successes and failures are also his own. The normal way to gain respect and advance himself is to enhance some of the great purposes of his department. And great purposes usually cost money.[34]

This points towards an economic theory of bureaucracy, and it does not appear unreasonable to assume that given the propensity to serve in a particular office for what often seems to be no more than a few months, senior Ministers would wish to have some tangible evidence of their impact upon policy even if, in the present economic climate, the claim is no more than that they successfully averted expenditure cuts demanded by the Treasury. For similar reasons, junior Ministers, though often closer to the details of individual plans and proposals, may be disinclined to invest in areas where credit is shared. In general, therefore joint 'planning' will only get off the ground where there is a strong political will in more than one Department. This is not surprising: for social policy is about conflict, and joint planning may be the unwilling victim.

Once again, however, any tentative steps taken at a national level towards a co-ordinated strategic approach could still founder at the level where social policies result in services, at the local level. Sceptics would cite that all the problems at Whitehall are replicated within local authorities and in their relationships with other bodies, not least health authorities. Others, with tempered optimism, might look to increasing attempts within local authorities towards corporate styles of management and believe that more joint planning at national levels would be a positive stimulus to local joint approaches to social policies.

The DHSS response to the latter view was a Health/Local Authority Consultative Circular[35] recommending arrangements for joint planning of complementary health and local authority services; and for joint financing of projects which have been planned jointly by health and local authorities. Through the Circular the Secretary of State encourages collaboration in planning between health and local authorities so that each authority contributes to all stages of the other's planning, from the first steps in developing common policies and strategies to the production of operational plans to carry them out. The Circular continues: 'only by full collaborative planning of this kind will health and local authorities feel equally committed to joint plans', though is noticeably silent in identifying the necessary and sufficient conditions for its success.

Certainly, at the time of writing, the desirability of joint planning is apparently less in question than is its feasibility. A key feature of the reorganisation of the NHS was the emphasis placed upon the need for effective collaboration between health and local authorities, and the principle of coterminous authority boundaries was designed to facilitate collaboration on both the planning and the operational delivery of services. There is little doubt that services provided by local authorities have a considerable impact on health services, and vice versa. But the issue goes deeper than this, for different services might indeed be substitutes for each other, which might upset the cosy assumptions made so far that their respective services are complementary and interlocking. The logic of this might be to allow priorities to be determined locally, by members and officers of both authorities deciding for themselves the most appropriate mix of services in the light of their local conditions and needs. Such a 'radical' strategy might, however, not only be contrary to the wishes of the central authorities in terms of the powers they wish to devolve but depend, once again, in turn upon the willingness of the respective local agencies to relinquish a degree of autonomy.

What limited evidence exists tends to suggest that all the emphasis to date has been upon establishing planning links between social service departments (LA) and the NHS, particularly in terms of the services they provide for such client groups as the elderly, mentally ill and handicapped. Yet, personal social services have equally important links with other local authority services (notably education and housing) which restrict their ability to act independently, as well as with other agencies outside local authorities (such as social security, probation services, employment services) and other community, often voluntary organisations. Equally, collaboration is not only dependent upon willingness to share ideas and goals at a political and administrative level but also upon the agreement of professionals at field level, between GP and social worker, between social worker and health visitor. This stage is the most vital, for it is here that social policy manifests itself in service by its degree of interprofessional co-ordination and co-operation.

Whether the sense of political autonomy of the local authority and the independence of its officers can be compromised with the carrot of 'joint financing' remains to be seen, but arrangements have been made to allow limited uses of resources available to health authorities for the purpose of supporting selected projects for which local authorities bear the prime responsibility. It must be recorded that the scheme is not universally highly rated, particularly as in some health circles there is regret that this represents a further earmarking of funds and evidence of centralised decision-making. Local authorities, for their part, feel aggrieved believing that, without the scheme they might have received the money direct, and that this really represents a further central grant to local authorities. The very fact that the implementation of schemes is entirely at the discretion of local authorities tends to support this hypothesis. The proposals for joint financing also allow a further speculation: namely, if the philosophy of community care (as opposed to hospital care) gains momentum, the 'seed money' to local authorities will need to be increased until the point is reached when a major new financing source occurs through subvention from health authorities. If this is not too fanciful an idea would this be the time when the case for placing health under local government[36] (or social services under health) becomes a politically viable proposition?

Some Concluding Thoughts

This essay opened with considerations of public expenditure and this concluding section first returns to this theme. In the DHSS working manual 'The NHS Planning System', issued to health authorities, planning is defined as 'deciding how the future pattern of activities should differ from the present, identifying the changes necessary to accomplish this, and specifying how these changes should be brought about'.[37] Whether fortuitous or not, the emphasis upon change and not growth is significant in the context in which the NHS now finds itself. Political parties in the House of Commons appear united in their wish to abate the pace of growth in public spending, albeit from different standpoints and for different purposes. Public expenditure has for long been a tool of economic policy; what makes it different this time round for the NHS is that the debate has shifted more noticeably towards policies on hospital closures. It is, of course, argued that the economic conditions now facing the UK, and likely to be present for some years to come, heighten the questions about the goals and priorities of the NHS, and therefore create the opportunity to seek a more efficient and equitable NHS. Yet, simultaneously, these very changes in our economic life-style, coupled with the upheaval created by reorganisation of the NHS structure itself, make both the introduction of the new NHS planning system and new policy initiatives difficult questions, and their acceptance an even more precarious business.

In the first place, the response to the health care challenge has been conceived in largely structural terms, both with regard to the reorganisation of the NHS itself and in the formulation of the NHS planning system. In that sense, the holistic approach — of comprehensive and corporate planning[38] — may have been too readily and eagerly accepted, in appearing to offer a seemingly rational solution to health care. Above all else, planning is about judgements, and frameworks and systems can be no more than enabling frameworks within which interested parties conduct their dialogue and ultimately reach their decisions. Certainly, the theory of joint planning is undoubtedly attractive in as much as the more comprehensively those in large organisations seek to plan, the more they find themselves dependent upon the outcomes of other agencies, whether public or private. Yet, comprehensive planning systems conceived in times of growth — when collaboration, co-operation and co-ordination between individuals and agencies could be more easily accommodated — is quite untried in times of financial stringency. Necessarily there are constraints imposed by the respective organisations within which their members and officers are obliged to operate. The provision of complementary health and social welfare services then depends upon the willingness of health and local authorities to modify their aspirations and, more crucially, expenditure patterns; where this willingness is not forthcoming, comprehensive health planning must be rendered less effective.

In the past criticisms have been directed at government of too much 'global' control aimed at economic management and too little 'detailed' analysis of individual policies. From that point of view it is doubtless true that wide variations exist in resource inputs, utilisation of services, and expenditure *per capita* between health (and local) authorities, and that Ministers have a ready-made opportunity to reap a high return on publicity from promulgating policies aimed at redressing these inequalities. Yet the dual notions of equity and equality are difficult to apply, for there is no consensus as to how they should be interpreted or, indeed, reconciled. Equity is more a matter of opinion than the automatic application of an incontrovertible principle; justice, fairness, equity, like beauty, ultimately lie in the eye of the beholder — or rather the receiver. The debate is far from over, for as time goes on and cuts begin to 'bite' it will require a fine judgement to decide how much redistribution is administratively possible and politically acceptable.

On another level the new initiatives in health planning at national and local levels are encouraging signs, though the lesson to be quickly learned here is that no one will sustain an interest in planning if it is allowed to lapse into a data chase, or a management game of paper plans incapable of being translated into reality. Model or utopian comprehensive health planning logically entails collecting an infinity of relevant data, and coding the whole constellation of human values into some universally agreed solution. Neither individuals nor organisations could comply with these requirements. Yet, any proposed system has to respond to the considerations raised in the comprehensive model. A key factor will be whether management will accept a modified comprehensive model with processes which are analytical and explicit, or whether it will find more comfort in its traditional unco-ordinated, incremental and intuitive approaches to real-life problems.

Finally, the major recurring theme through this essay has been the interplay between central government and local agencies. The key to the changing shape of central — local relations is the disposition of government to accelerate the trend towards centralisation — and is not each central initiative accompanied by expression of severe regret — and the strength of resistance of local bodies to the trend. Whether local democracy is threatened — by no means a novel theme in political writings over the last century — is debatable, particularly as evidence to demonstrate uniformity of levels of service throughout the country is hard to come by. A consistent half-way position in the centralist — localist controversy is likely to prove elusive, if only because half-way positions depend upon those taken at the extremities and these can be reliably estimated to be different from one issue to another. Like the poor, this particular conflict is with us always. The NHS will just have to live with the paradox that it operates on too large a scale for it to be easily amenable to close central management; yet at the same time the fact that it is big business, its claims on public expenditure, and its political importance makes it an automatic candidate for central control. It is also such tensions as these together with others revealed in this series of essays that make the NHS the inevitable periodic if not perennial subject for Royal Commissions.

Notes

1. See, for instance, R. Maxwell, *'Health Care: The Growing Dilemma'*, 2nd edition, McKinsey, New York, 1975; D. Macmillan, 'The Infinity of Demand: A Case for Integration' in *NHS Reorganisation: Issues and Prospects*, edited by K. Barnard and K. Lee, University of Leeds, 1974; Office of Health Economics, *The Health Care Dilemma*, August 1975.
2. DHSS Circular, *National Health Service Planning System*, HSC (IS) 126, March 1975.
3. The Department is sponsoring a research programme covering the introduction and early years of operation of the NHS planning system. The research is being conducted in selected Regions, Areas and Districts by three commissioned research teams, the editors of this book being co-directors of one such team. See HC (76) 30, *Health Services Management. The NHS Planning System: Planning Activity in 1976/77*, June 1976.
4. A. Crosland, 'The battle for the public purse', *Guardian*, 24 March 1976, the text of a Fabian Lecture delivered the same day.
5. HMSO, *Public Expenditure to 1979-80*, Cmnd. 6393, February 1976.
6. Though this description is delightfully vague, it is as well to be so in an economic climate where White Papers, unlike their predecessors, barely retain credibility over the next four months, let alone the next four years.
7. Notably by Mr Wynne Godley of the University of Cambridge, Department of Applied Economics, and a former deputy director of the Treasury's economic sector.
8. R. Klein, *et al.*, *Constraints and Choices*, Centre for Studies in Social Policy, March 1976.
9. H. Glennerster, 'In Praise of Public Expenditure', *New Statesman*, 27 February 1976, puts it more vividly: 'the vision of the social services stage coach, driven by local authority treasurer bandits, careering along wildly out of control, is even further from the truth than most westerns.'
10. HMSO, *Cash Limits on Public Expenditure*, Cmnd. 6440, April 1976.
11. A principal exclusion from cash limits in 1976/7 is the cost of family practitioner services which remain predominantly open-ended commitments least capable of firm financial control. These at present account for over one-fifth of the NHS budget and, somewhat ironically, it is in this very area where the government is proposing a major expenditure growth over the next few years.
12. See D. Lees, 'Economics and Non-Economics of Health Services', *Three Banks Review*, June 1976, p. 20.
13. HMSO, *Local Government Finance;* Report of the Committee of Inquiry, Cmnd. 6453, May 1976. Chairman, Sir Frank Layfield, Q.C.
14. The article by A. Crispin, 'Local Government Finance: Assessing the Central Government's Contribution', *Public Administration*, Spring 1976, represents a recent attempt to establish the level of government's financial support to the totality of local authority expenditure.
15. Professor Alan Day takes issue with his colleagues on the Layfield Committee in seeking to explain the growth of centrally funded expenditure. In a *Note of Reservation* he states— 'I would lay more emphasis than the Report on causation running from political aims and policies to finance mechanisms, rather than in the opposite direction', p. 306 and 'the rising proportion of government grants has primarily been the consequence (rather than the cause) of a growing desire of the government to achieve rapid rise in the standards of local government services', p. 303.
16. For further details see *Local Government Finance*, Annex 27.
17. P. Townsend, 'Area Deprivation Policies', *New Statesman*, 6 August 1976,

p. 170, was prepared to go further—'but it would be wrong to suppose that resources are allocated substantially in accordance with any reasonable definition of needs. In practice many of the indicators of need are crudely defined and are weighted by a piece of technical wizardry which obscures the bureaucratic conservatism of the exercise'.

18. D. Pyle, 'Aspects of Resource Allocation by Local Education Authorities', *Social and Economic Administration,* Summer 1976, writes: 'There is quite considerable scope for autonomy on the part of LEAs in deciding on educational policy...not only on matters of style...but also in terms of the amount of resources used in the education services,' p. 111.

19. DHSS Circular LASSL (75) 3, *Local Authorities Social Services Capital Programme. Secretary of State's List of Schemes Selected for 1975/76.* In explaining the process by which LAs social services capital schemes gained approval for 1975/6 the then Secretary of State stated: 'In a small number of cases a scheme has been included although the local authority concerned gave it lower priority than another scheme which has been omitted. They have been included because...the Secretary of State suggests that, in order to ensure fulfilment in 1975/6 of a mental illness programme of the scale local authorities, taken together, clearly intend, it will be desirable for planning of these schemes to go ahead side by side with the planning of the schemes of higher priority.'

20. DHSS, *Priorities for Health and Personal Social Services in England: A Consultative Document,* 1976.

21. Thus, for example, it is estimated that at present there are approximately six home helps per 1,000 elderly whereas the national guideline is for 12 per 1,000. Given the national target suggested for expanding home helps is 2 per cent a year the picture will hardly change overnight—indeed the guideline will only be capable of being met well into the next century.

22. For instance, M. J. Buxton and R. E. Klein, 'Distribution of Hospital Provision: Policy Themes and Resource Variations', *British Medical Journal,* 8 February 1975; A. H. Snaith, 'Regional Variations in the Allocation of Financial Resources to the Community Health Service', *The Lancet,* 30 March 1974; P. H. Gentle and J. M. Forsythe, 'Revenue Allocation in the Reorganised Health Service', *BMJ,* 9 August 1975; J. H. Rickard, 'Per capita expenditure of the English area health authorities', *BMJ,* 31 January 1976.

23. DHSS, *First Interim Report of the Resource Allocation Working Party,* August 1975.

24. HMSO, *Sharing Resources for Health in England,* report of the Resource Allocation Working Party, September 1976.

25. 'Equality' as a notion is hard to pin down. For some recent attempts see J. Vaizey, [ed], *Whatever happened to equality?,* British Broadcasting Corporation, 1975.

26. J. Butler, 'How many doctors are needed in general practice?' *BMJ,* 17 January 1976.

27. For an exploration of these issues see P. Townsend, 'Inequality and the Health Service', *The Lancet,* 15 June 1974.

28. P. Townsend, 'Area Deprivation Policies', op. cit., p. 170.

29. The concept of 'access' is more problematic than might at first sight appear. See R. Fein, 'On Achieving Access and Equity in Health Care', *MMFQ,* October 1972; L. A. Aday, and R. Anderson, *Access to Medical Care,* Health Administration Press, 1975.

30. A. Cartwright and M. O'Brien, 'Social Class Variations in Health Care and in the Nature of General Practitioner Consultations', in M. Stacey, [ed], *The Sociology of the NHS,* Sociological Review Monograph, March 1976, p. 84.

31. See S. Holtermann, 'Areas of urban deprivation in Great Britain: an analysis of 1971 Census data', *CSO Social Trends*, No. 6, HMSO, 1975.
32. HMSO, *A Joint Framework for Social Policy*, June 1975.
33. R. Bourne, 'Joint social policy—or crowns and courtiers', *New Society*, 27 November 1975.
34. H. Heclo and A. Wildavsky, *The Private Government of Public Money*, Macmillan, 1974, pp. 134-5.
35. DHSS, *Joint Care Planning: Health and Local Authorities*, Circular HC(76)18, March 1976.
36. Ironically, it would appear that a section of the general public already believe this to be the case. For example, the Layfield Committee, in commissioning a survey of public attitudes to local government, found that 54 per cent of those interviewed thought hospitals were supplied by LAs, wholly or partly from the rates, p. 9.
37. DHSS, *The NHS Planning System*, Working Manual, May 1976, p. 5.
38. For a flavour of the UK debate see P. Self, 'Is Comprehensive Planning Possible and Rational?', *Policy and Politics*, Vol. 2, No. 3, 1974; and B. Taylor, 'Strategies for Planning', *Long Range Planning*, August 1975.

BIBLIOGRAPHY

Publications

Abel-Smith, B., and Gales,K., *British Doctors at Home and Abroad,* Occasional Papers on Social Administration, No. 8, Bell and Sons, London, 1962.

Abel-Smith, B., *Value for Money in Health Services,* Heinemann, London, 1976.

ACAHA, *A Review of the Management of the Reorganised NHS,* Working Party of the Association of Chief Administrators of Health Authorities, 1975.

Acheson, R. M., 'Basic and Continuing Education of Community Physicians', *Health Trends,* 7, 1975.

Aday, L. A., and Anderson, R., *Access to Medical Care,* Health Administration Press, 1975.

Aldridge, L. W., 'The Organisation and Staffing of Casualty Departments', *Postgraduate Medical Journal,* Vol. 48, 1972.

Ashworth, W., and Mitchell, G., 'The CHC and its Public', *The Hospital and Health Services Review,* June 1976.

Bachrach, P., and Baratz, M. S., *Power and Poverty,* Oxford University Press, New York, 1970.

Baderman, H., 'Accident and Emergency Services', *Kings Fund Centre Reprint No. 945,* 1975.

Barnard, K., and Lee, K. (eds.), *NHS Reorganisation: Issues and Prospects,* University of Leeds, 1974.

Barnard, K., and Ham, C., 'The Reallocation of Resources: Parallels with Past Experience', *The Lancet,* 26 June 1976.

Barron, R., and Norris, G., 'Sexual Divisions and the Dual Labour Market', in D. Leonard Barker and S. Allen (eds.)., *Dependence and Exploitation in Work and Marriage,* Longmans, London, 1976.

Bastide, R., 'Prolegomena to a Sociology of Mental Disorder' in *The Sociology of Mental Disorder,* Routledge and Kegan Paul, London, 1972.

Bayley, M., *Mental Handicap and Community Care,* Routledge and Kegan Paul, London 1973.

Becker, H. S., *et al.* (eds.), 'Boys in White', *Student Culture in the Medical School,* University of Chicago Press, Chicago, 1961.

Becker, H. S., *et al.* (eds.), *Institutions and the Person,* Aldine, Chicago, 1968.

Beer, S. H., *Modern British Politics,* Faber, London, 2nd edition, 1969.

Belmar, R., and Sidel, V. W., 'An International Perspective on Strikes and Strike Threats by Physicians: the case of Chile', *International Journal of Health Services,* 5, 1, 1975.

Bentley, A. F., *The Process of Government,* Harvard University Press, Cambridge, 1967 (first published 1908).

Bevan, A., *In Place of Fear,* MacGibbon and Kee, London, 1961.

Birch, A. H., *Representative and Responsible Government,* Allen and Unwin, London, 1964.

BMA, *Accident Services of Great Britain and Ireland,* British Medical Association, 1965.

Blalock, H. M., *Social Statistics,* McGraw-Hill, 1970.

Bloom, S. W., 'The Process of Becoming a Physician', *The Annals of the American Academy of Political and Social Science,* Vol. 346, March 1963.

Bloor, M., and Horobin, G., 'Conflict and Conflict Resolution in Doctor/Patient Interactions' in C. Cox and A. Meade (eds.), *A Sociology of Medical Practice,* Collier-Macmillan, London, 1975.

BOA, *Casualty Departments—The Accident Commitment,* British Orthopaedic Association, 1973.

Bourne, R., 'Joint Social Policy—or crowns and courtiers', *New Society,* 27 November 1975.

Boyle, C. M., 'Differences between Patients' and Doctors' Interpretations of some common Medical Terms', *BMJ,* May 1970.

Brannen, P., *et al., The Worker Directors,* Hutchinson, London, 1976.

Brass, W., 'On the Possibility of Population Prediction' in C. Freeman, M. Jahoda and I. Miles, *Progress and Problems in Social Forecasting,* SSRC, 1972.

Brass, W., 'Perspectives in Population Prediction; illustrated by the statistics of England and Wales', *Journal of the Royal Statistical Society,* Series A., Vol. 137, 1974.

Bridger, H., Mars, G., Miller, E., Scott, S., and Towell, D., *An Exploratory Study of the RCN Membership Structure,* Royal College of Nursing, London, 1973.

Brown, R. G. S., *The Management of Welfare,* Fontana, London 1975.

Brown, R. G. S., Griffin, S., and Haywood, S. C., *New Bottles: Old Wine?,* Institute for Health Studies, University of Hull, 1975.

Bruggen, P., and Bourne, S., 'Further Examination of the Distinction Awards System in England and Wales', *BMJ,* 28 February 1976.

Bucher, R., and Strauss, A., 'Professions in Process', *American Journal of Sociology,* 66, 1961.

Burnley, R. E., and Sadler, A. M., 'Resources Utilised for the Care of Surgical Patients in the Emergency Department', *Medical Care,* December 1975.

Butler, J. R., 'Illness and the Sick Role: An Evaluation in Three Communities', *British Journal of Sociology,* Vol. 21, 3 September 1970.

Butler, J., 'How many doctors are needed in general practice?', *BMJ,* 17 January 1976.

Butler, Samuel, *Erewhon,* Penguin Books, Harmondsworth, 1970 (first published 1872).

Buxton, M. J., and Klein, R.E., 'Distribution of Hospital Provision: Policy Themes and Resource Variations', *BMJ,* 8 February 1975.

Buxton, M., and Craven, E. (eds.), *Demographic Change and Social Policy: The Uncertain Future,* Centre for Studies in Social Policy, London, September 1976.

Caro, D. B., 'The Casualty Surgeons Association', *Postgraduate Medical Journal,* Vol. 48, 1972.

Carr-Saunders, A. M., and Wilson, P. A., *The Professions,* Oxford University Press, Oxford, 1933.

Cartwright, A., *Human Relations and Hospital Care,* Routledge and Kegan Paul, London, 1967.

Cartwright, A., *Patients and their Doctors,* Routledge and Kegan Paul, London, 1967.

Cartwright, A., *How Many Children,* Routledge and Kegan Paul, London, 1976.

Cartwright, A., and O'Brien, M., 'Social Class Variations in Health Care and in the Nature of General Practitioner Consultations' in M. Stacey (ed.), *The Sociology of the NHS,* Sociological Review Monograph 22, March 1976.

Casualty Surgeons Association, *An Integrated Emergency Service,* Casualty Surgeons Association, 1973.

Christiansen, U., 'Demand for Emergency Health Care and Regional Systems for Provision of Supply' in M. Perlman (ed.), *The Economics of Health and Medical Care,* 1974.

Clarke, R. O., Fatchett, D. J., and Roberts, B. C., *Workers' Participation in Management in Britain,* Heinemann, London, 1972.

Clegg, H. A., and Chester, T. E., *Wage Policy and the Health Service,* Basil Blackwell, Oxford, 1957.

Clegg, H. A., *A New Approach to Industrial Democracy,* Blackwell, Oxford, 1960.

Cobb, B., 'Why do Patients de-tour to Quacks?' in E. G. Jaco (ed.), *Patients, Physicians and Illness,* Free Press, New York, 1958.

Cochrane, A. L., *Effectiveness and Efficiency: Random Reflections on Health Services*, Nuffield Provincial Hospitals Trust, London, 1972.

Coe, Rodney, *Sociology of Medicine*, McGraw-Hill, New York, 1970.

Community Relations Commission, *Doctors from Overseas: A Case for Consultation*, London, 1976.

Conway, H., 'Emergency Medical Care', *BMJ*, 28 August 1976.

Cowan, L., and Cowan, M., *The Wit of Medicine*, Leslie Frewin, London, 1972.

Cox, C., and Meade, A. (eds.), *A Sociology of Medical Practice*, Collier-Macmillan, London, 1975.

Crispin, A., 'Local Government Finance: Assessing the Central Government's Contribution', *Public Administration*, Spring 1976.

Crombie, D. L., 'A Casualty Survey', *Journal of the College of General Practitioners*, Vol. 2, 1959.

Cross, D. T., 'Planning Forecasting' in C. Freeman, M. Jahoda and I. Miles, *Progress and Problems in Social Forecasting*, SSRC, 1972.

Cross, P., 'Population Analysis in Hackney', *Greater London Intelligence Quarterly*, No. 30, 1975.

Cull, T., 'The General Practitioners' View', *Postgraduate Medical Journal*, Vol. 48, 1972.

Cummings, G., 'The role of the clinician in the reorganised NHS— an eye witness account', *Hospital and Health Services Review*, 6, 72, and 7, 72, 1976.

Dahl, R. A., *A Preface to Democratic Theory*, University of Chicago, Chicago, 1956.

Dahl, R. A., *Who Governs?*, Yale University Press, New Haven, 1961.

Dahl, R. A., *Pluralist Democracy in the United States*, Rand McNally, Chicago, 1967.

Dartington, T., and Miller, E. J., *Geriatric Hospital Care*, Tavistock Institute for Human Relations, London, 1975.

Davies, C., 'Professionals in Organisations: some preliminary observations on hospital consultants', *Sociological Review*, 20, 4, 1972.

Davis, F., *Passage Through Crisis: Polio Victims and Their Families*, Bobbs-Merrill, Indianapolis, 1962.

Davis, N. H. W., 'Population Projections: The Certainty of the Uncertain Future' in M. Buxton and E. Craven (eds.), *Demographic Change and Social Policy: The Uncertain Future*, Centre for Studies in Social Policy, London, September 1976.

Davis, N., 'Britain's Changing Age Structure 1971-2011', *Population Trends*, No. 3, Spring 1976.

De Finetti, B., 'Foresight: Its Logical Laws, Its Subjective Sources'

(1937) in H. E. Kyburg and H. E. Smokler, *Studies in Subjective Probability,* Wiley, 1964.

De Finetti, B., *Theory of Probability: A Critical Introductory Treatment,* Vol. 1, Wiley, London, 1974.

Dickinson, C. W., and Hodgetts, I. R., 'Participation in Practice', *Health and Social Services Journal,* 18 October 1975.

Dimmock, S. J., and Farnham, D., 'Working with Whitley in Today's NHS', *Personnel Management,* January 1975.

Doran, F. S. A., 'Expansion of the Consultant Grade', *BMJ,* 10 March 1973.

Dorn, H. F., 'Pitfalls in Population Forecasts and Projections', *Journal of the American Statistical Association,* Vol.45, No. 251, 1950.

Draper, P., and Smart, T., 'Social Science and Health Policy in the United Kingdom: Some Contributions of the Social Sciences to the Bureaucratisation of the National Health Service', *International Journal of Health Services,* 4 (3), 1974.

Draper, P., Greenholm, G., and Best, G., 'The Organisation of Health Care: A Critical View of the 1974 Reorganisation of the National Health Service' in D. Tuckett (ed.), *Introduction to Medical Sociology,* Tavistock, London, 1976.

Draper, P., Best, G., and Dennis, J., *Health, Money and the National Health Service,* Unit for the Study of Health Policy, Department of Community Medicine, Guy's Hospital Medical School, 1976.

Dunnell, K., and Cartwright, A., *Medicine Takers, Prescribers and Hoarders,* Routledge and Kegan Paul, London, 1972.

Dyson, R. F., *Ancillary Staff Industrial Action, Spring 1973,* Leeds Regional Hospital Board, Leeds, 1974.

Eckstein, H., *The English Health Service: its origins, structures and achievements,* Harvard Unit Press, Cambridge, Massachusetts, 1958.

Eckstein, H., *Pressure Group Politics,* Allen and Unwin, London, 1960.

Emery, F. E., and Thorsrud, E., *Form and Content in Industrial Democracy,* Tavistock Publications, London, 1969.

Fein, R., 'On Achieving Access and Equity in Health Care', *MMFQ,* October 1972.

Fellner, W., *Probability and Profit,* Irwin, Homewood, Illinois, 1965.

Fenn, M., Mungovan, R., and Towell, D., 'Developing the Role of the Unit Nursing Officer', *Nursing Times,* 71, 1975.

Finer, S. E., 'The Political Power of Organised Labour', *Government and Opposition,* Vol. 8, 1973.

Forsyth, G., *Doctors and State Medicine,* Pitman Medical, London, 1966.

Foot, M., *Aneurin Bevan, 1945-60*, Paladin, London, 1975.

Fox, A., 'Industrial Sociology and Industrial Relations, Research Paper No. 3', *Royal Commission on Trade Unions and Employers' Associations*, HMSO, London, 1966.

Fox, A., 'A Social Critique of Pluralist Ideology' in J. Child (ed.), *Man and Organisation*, George Allen and Unwin, London, 1973.

Fox, A., *Beyond Contract: Work, Power and Trust Relations*, Faber and Faber, London, 1974.

Freidson, E., *Patients' Views of Medical Practice*, Russell Sage, New York, 1961.

Freidson, E., *Professional Dominance: The Social Structure of Medical Care*, Atherton, New York, 1972.

Freidson, E., *Profession of Medicine: A Study of the Sociology of Applied Knowledge*, Dodd Mead, New York, 1970.

French, J. P. R., Jnr., *et al.*, 'An experiment on participation in a Norwegian factory', *Human Relations*, Vol. 13, 1960.

Friend, J., Power, J., and Yewlett, C., *Public Planning: The Intercorporate Dimension*, Tavistock, London, 1974.

Furstenberg, F., 'Workers' Participation in Management in the Federal Republic of Germany', *International Institute for Labour Studies*, Bulletin 6, 1969.

Gentle, P. H., and Forsythe, J. M., 'Revenue Allocation in the Reorganised.Health Service', *BMJ*, 9 August 1975.

Georgopoulos, B. S., and Matijko, A., 'The American General Hospital as a Complex Social System', *Health Services Research*, Spring 1967.

Gill, D. G., 'The British National Health Service: Professional determinants of administrative structure', *International Journal of Health Services*, 1, 4, 1971.

Gill, D. G., 'The Reorganisation of the National Health Service: Some Sociological Aspects with special reference to the role of the Community Physician' in M. Stacey (ed.), *The Sociology of the National Health Service*, Sociological Review Monograph No. 22, 1976.

Gish, O., *Doctor Migration and World Health*, Occasional Papers in Social Administration, No. 43, Bell and Sons, London, 1971.

Glass, D. V., 'Demographic Prediction', *Proceedings of the Royal Society of London*, Series B., Vol. 168, 1967.

Glass, D. V., 'The History of Population Forecasting' in C. Freeman, M. Jahoda and I. Miles, *Progress and Problems in Social Forecasting*, SSRC, 1972.

Glennerster, H., 'In Praise of Public Expenditure', *New Statesman*, 27 February 1976.

Godber, G., *The Health Service: Past, Present and Future,* The Athlone Press, University of London, 1975.

Goffman, E., *Asylums,* Penguin, Harmondsworth, 1961.

Goffman, E., *Interaction Ritual,* Penguin University Books, Harmondsworth, 1972.

Goldthorpe, J. H., *et al., The Affluent Worker in the Class Structure,* Cambridge University Press, Cambridge, 1969.

Goldsen, R. K., *et al.,* 'Some factors related to Patient Delay in Seeking Diagnosis for Cancer Symptoms', *Cancer,* 10, 1, January-February 1957.

Golembiewski, R. T., *Organising Men and Power: patterns of behaviour and line-staff models,* Rand McNally and Co., Chicago, 1967.

Goode, W. J., 'Community Within a Community: The Professions', *American Sociological Review,* Vol. 22, April 1957.

Gostin, L., *A Human Condition: The Mental Health Act 1959-1975,* MIND, 1975.

Green, S., *The Hospital: An Organisation Analysis,* Blackie, Glasgow, 1974.

Green, S., 'Professional/Bureaucratic Conflict: The Case of the Medical Profession in the National Health Service', *Sociological Review,* 1, 23, February 1975.

Gruenberg, E. M., 'The Future of Community Medicine', *The Lancet,* 31 July 1976.

Hall, R., 'Professionalization and Bureaucratization', *American Sociological Review,* Vol. 33, February 1968.

Hallas, J., *Mounting the Health Guard: A Handbook for Community Health Councils,* Nuffield Provincial Hospitals Trust, London, 1974.

Hallas, J., *CHCs in Action,* Nuffield Provincial Hospitals Trust, London, 1976.

Harris, A., *The Handicapped and Impaired in Great Britain,* HMSO, 1973.

Heath, P. J., and Parry, W. H., 'Community Medicine: Has it a future?', *The Lancet,* 9 July 1976.

Heclo, H., and Wildavsky, A., *The Private Government of Public Money,* Macmillan, 1974.

Hershey, N., 'The Defensive Practice of Medicine—Myth or Reality?', *Milbank Memorial Fund Quarterly,* 1972.

Hewitt, D., and Wood, P. H. N., 'Heterodox Practitioners and the Availability of Specialist Advice', *Rheumatology and Rehabilitation,* 14, 191, 1975.

High, D., McDowell, A., Meara, R., and Sharply, J., 'Hospitals and Industrial Relations', *British Hospital Journal and Social Science Review,*

Vol. 82, No. 2, 1972.

Hofstede, G., and Kassen, M. S. (eds.), *European Contributions to Organisation Theory,* Van Gorcum, Amsterdam, 1975.

Holtermann, S., 'Areas of Urban Deprivation in Great Britain: An Analysis of 1971 Census Data', *Social Trends,* No. 6, 1975.

Hughes, E. C., *Men and their Work,* Free Press, Glencoe, Illinois, 1958.

Hunter, T. D., 'Arena or amoeba: managing the health care network', *The Hospital,* April 1971.

IHA, *The Administration of the Hospital Service,* Institute of Hospital Administrators, 1951.

IHSA, *A Report on the Role of Unit and Sector Administrators in the National Health Service,* Institute of Health Service Administrators, 1976.

Illich, I., *Medical Nemesis: The Expropriation of Health,* Calder and Boyars, London, 1975.

Illich, I., *Limits to Medicine,* Marion Boyars, London, 1976.

Jerman, B., *Do Something: a guide to self-help organisations,* Garnstone Press, London, 1971.

Johnson, M.L., 'Self-Perception of Need Amongst the Elderly: An Analysis of Illness Behaviour', *Sociological Review,* Vol. 20, No. 4, November 1972.

Johnson, M.L., 'Whose Stranger Am I? Or, Patients Really Are People' in K. Barnard and K. Lee (eds.), *NHS Reorganisation: Issues and Prospects,* Nuffield Centre for Health Services Studies, University of Leeds, 1974.

Johnson, T.J., *Professions and Power,* Macmillan, London, 1972.

Joyce, C. R. B., 'Patient co-operation and the Sensitivity of Clinical Trials', *Journal of Chronic Diseases,* 15, 1962.

Kessell, W. I. N., 'The Psychiatric Morbidity in a London General Practice', *British Journal of Social and Preventive Medicine,* 14, 16, 1960.

Keyfitz, N., 'On Future Population', *Journal of the Statistical Association,* Vol. 67, No. 338, 1972.

Klarman, H. E., 'National Policies and Local Planning for Health Services', *Milbank Memorial Fund Quarterly,* Health and Society, Vol. 54, No. 4, 1975.

Klein, R., 'Health Services: The Case for A Counter-Bureaucracy', in S. Hatch (ed.), *Towards Participation in Local Services,* Fabian Tract. 419, 1973.

Klein, R., 'Policy Problems and Policy Perceptions in the National Health Service', *Policy and Politics,* Vol. 2, 1974.

Klein, R., 'Policy Making in the National Health Service', *Political*

Studies, Vol. 22, 1974.

Klein, R., *et al., Constraints and Choices,* Centre for Studies in Social Policy, March 1976.

Klein, R., and Lewis, J., *The Politics of Consumer Representation, A Study of Community Health Councils,* Centre for Studies in Social Policy, London, 1976.

Kohn, R., and White, K. L. (eds.), *Health Care: An International Study,* Oxford University Press, London, 1976.

Koos, E. L., *The Health of Regionville,* Hafner Publishing Co., New York, 1954.

Lammers, C. J., 'Power and participation in decision making in formal organisations', *American Journal of Sociology,* Vol. 73, No. 2, 1967.

Lees, D., 'Economics and Non-Economics of Health Services', *Three Banks Review,* June 1976.

Leif, H. I., *et al.* (eds.), *The Psychological Base of Medical Practice,* Harper and Row, New York, 1964.

Leighton, J., 'Primary Medical Care for the Homeless and Rootless in Liverpool', *Hospitals and Health Services Review,* August 1976.

Lewis A., 'Medicine and the Affections of the Mind', *BMJ,* 2, 1963.

Lipsky, M., 'Protest as a Political Resource', *American Political Science Review,* Vol. 62, 1968.

Lowden, T. G., 'The Casualty Department—The Work and the Staff', *The Lancet,* 16 June 1956.

Lowden, T. G., 'The Casualty Department—Shortcomings and Difficulties', *The Lancet,* 23 June 1956.

Lukes, S., *Power: A Radical View,* Macmillan, London 1974.

McCall, G. J., and Simmons, J. L., *Identities and Interactions,* Free Press, New York, 1966.

McCarthy, W. E. J., *The Role of Shop Stewards in British Industrial Relations,* Research Paper No. 1, Royal Commission on Trade Unions and Employers' Associations, HMSO, London, 1966.

Maclean, U., *Magical Medicine, A Nigerian Case Study,* Allen Lane, Penguin Press, London, 1973.

Maclean, U., 'Patient Delay: Some Observations on Medical Claims to Certainty', *The Lancet,* 23, 5 July 1975.

McDermott, S., 'Analysing the need for paramedics', *The Journal of Emergency Care and Transportation,* 5, 2, 1976.

McKenzie, R., and Silver, A., *Angels in Marble,* Heinemann, London, 1968.

McKeown, T., *A Historical Appraisal of the Medical Task,* in G. McLachlan and T. McKeown (eds.), *Medical History and Medical Care,*

Nuffield Provincial Hospitals Trust, Oxford, 1971.

McKinlay, J. B., 'On the Professional Regulation of Change', in P. Halmos (ed.), *Professionalisation and Social Change*, Sociological Review Monograph, No.20, 1973.

McLachlan, G. (ed.), *In Low Gear? An Examination of Cogwheels*, Nuffield Provincial Hospitals Trust, London, 1971.

Macmillan, D., 'The Infinity of Demand: A Case for Integration' in *NHS Reorganisation: Issues and Prospects*, K. Barnard and K. Lee (eds.), University of Leeds, 1974.

Marmor, T., and Thomas, D., 'Doctors, Politics and Pay Disputes', *British Journal of Political Science*, Vol. 2, 1972.

Marsh, A. I., and Coker, E., 'Shop Steward Organisation in Engineering', *British Journal of Industrial Relations*, Vol. 1, No. 2, 1973.

Maxwell, R., *Health Care: The Growing Dilemma*, 2nd edition, McKinsey, New York, 1975.

Mechanic, D., 'The Concept of Illness Behaviour', *Journal of Chronic Diseases*, 15, 1961.

Mechanic, D., *Medical Sociology, A Selective View*, Free Press, Glencoe, Illinois, 1968.

Mechanic, D., 'Correlates of Frustration among British General Practitioners', *Journal of Health and Social Behaviour*, 11, 2, 1970.

Merton, R. K., *et al.*, *The Student Physician*, Harvard University Press, Cambridge, Massachusetts, 1957.

Miles, A. W., and Smith, D., *Joint Consultation: Defeat or Opportunity?*, Kings Fund, London, 1969.

Miliband, R., *The State in Capitalist Society*, Quartet, London, 1973.

Mills, G., and Howe, M., 'Consumer Representation and the Withdrawal of Railway Services', *Public Administration*, Vol. 38, 1960.

Murphy, F. W., 'District Community Physician-Activity Analysis', *Public Health London*, 89, 1975.

Navarro, V., 'The Political Economy of Health Care: An explanation of the composition, nature, and functions of the present health sector of the United States', *Institute of Health Services*, 5, 1, 1975.

Navarro, V., 'Women in Health Care', *New England Journal of Medicine*, Vol. 229, No. 8, 1975.

Newby, H., 'The Deferential Dialectic', *Comparative Studies in History and Society*, 17, 2, April 1975.

Newton, K., 'A Critique of the Pluralist Model', *Acta Sociologica*, Vol. 12, 1969.

Nightingale, B., *Charities*, Allen Lane, London, 1973.

Nordlinger, E. A., *The Working Class Tories*, McGibbon and Kee,

London, 1967.

Nuffield Provincial Hospitals Trust, *Casualty Services and Their Settings,* Oxford University Press, 1960.

Nuffield Provincial Hospitals Trust, *Ninth Report 1970-1975,* Nuffield Provincial Hospitals Trust, 1975.

Office of Health Economics, *The Health Care Dilemma,* August 1975.

Owen, D., 'Clinical Freedom and Professional Freedom', *The Lancet,* 8 May 1976.

Parkhouse, J., 'Medical Manpower', *The Lancet,* 11 September 1976.

Parry, N., and Parry, J., 'The Teacher and Professionalism: the failure of an occupational strategy' in M. Flude and J. Ahier, *Educability, Schools and Ideology,* Croom Helm, London, 1974.

Parry, N., and Parry, J., *The Rise of the Medical Profession,* Croom Helm, London, 1976.

Parsons, T., *The Social System,* Free Press, Glencoe, Illinois, 1951.

Patel, A. R., 'Modes of Admission to Hospital: A Survey of Emergency Admissions to General Medical Unit', *BMJ,* 30 January 1971.

Patey, D. G. H., 'The District Community Physician in Practice', *Health Trends,* 7, 1975.

Pearce, D., 'Births and Family Formation Patterns', *Population Trends,* No. 1, 1975.

Pease, R., 'A Study of Patients in a London Accident and Emergency Department', *The Practitioner,* Vol. 211, November 1973.

Peel, J., 'The Hull Family Survey', *Journal of Bio Social Science,* 1970, 1972.

Peel, J., and Carr, G., *Contraception and Family Design,* Churchill Livingstone, Edinburgh, 1975.

Petrie, A., *Individuality in Pain and Suffering,* University of Chicago Press, Chicago, 1967.

Plant, R., *Community and Ideology,* Routledge and Kegan Paul, London, 1974.

Powles, J., 'On the Limitations of Modern Medicine', *Social Science and Man,* 1, 1973.

Pyle, D., 'Aspects of Resource Allocation by Local Education Authorities', *Social and Economic Administration,* Summer 1976.

Raphael, W., *Patients and Their Hospitals,* King Edward's Hospital Fund for London, London, 1969.

Rickard, J. H., 'Per capita expenditure of the English area health authorities', *BMJ,* 31 January 1976.

Roberts, N., *Our Future Selves,* Allen and Unwin, London, 1970.

Robinson, D., *The Process of Becoming Ill,* Routledge and Kegan Paul,

London, 1971.

Roth, J., *Timetables: Structuring the Passage of Time in Hospital and Other Careers,* Bobbs-Merrill, Indanapolis, 1963.

Royal College of Physicians, *A Review of the Medical Services in Great Britain,* London, 1962.

Runciman, W. G., *Relative Deprivation and Social Justice,* Routledge and Kegan Paul, London, 1966.

Ryder, N. B., and Westoff, C. F., *Reproduction in the United States, 1965,* Princetown University Press, 1971.

Saunders, L., *Cultural Difference and Medical Care,* Russell Sage, New York, 1954.

Schattschneider, E. E., *The Semi-Sovereign People,* Holt, Rinehart and Wilson, New York, 1960.

Scherer, J., *Contemporary Community,* Tavistock, London, 1972.

Schulman, S., and Smith, A. M., 'The Concept of Health Among Spanish Speaking Villagers of New Mexico and Colorado', *Journal of Health and Social Behaviour,* 4, Winter 1963.

Scott, W. H., *et al., Coal and Conflict: A Study of Industrial Relations at Collieries,* Liverpool University Press, 1963.

Scott, J. C., 'The Development of Accident Services: Accident and Emergency Services', *British Health Care and Technology,* Health and Social Services Journal/Hospital International, 1973.

Self, P., 'Is Comprehensive Planning Possible and Rational?', *Policy and Politics,* Vol. 2, No. 3, 1974.

Senewiratne, B., 'The Emigration of Doctors: A Problem for the Developing and the Developed Countries', *The Lancet,* 15 and 22 March 1975.

Shepherd, M., *et al., Psychiatric Illness in General Practice,* Oxford University Press, London, 1966.

Smith, L. R., 'From Ambulance Driver to EMT', *Hospitals,* Vol. 47, 16 May 1973.

Snaith, A. H., *et al.,* 'Regional Variations in the Allocation of Financial Resources to Community Health Service', *The Lancet,* 30 March 1974.

Spencer, J. A., 'Shaping Management in Oxfordshire', *Health and Social Service Journal,* 10 July 1976.

Stacey, M., *et al., Hospitals, Children and their Families,* Routledge and Kegan Paul, London, 1970.

Stacey, M. (ed.), *The Sociology of the NHS,* Sociological Review Monograph 22, Keele, March 1976.

Stevens, R., *Medical Practice in Modern England,* Yale University Press,

New Haven, 1966.

Stewart, M., *Unpaid Public Service,* Fabian Society, London, 1964.

Stimson, G., and Webb, B., *Going to See the Doctor, The Consultation Process in General Practice,* Routledge and Kegan Paul, 1975.

Strauss, A. L., *Mirrors and Masks,* Free Press, Glencoe, Illinois, 1959.

Strauss, A. L., *Psychiatric Ideologies and Institutions,* Free Press, Glencoe, Illinois, 1964.

Tannenbaum, A. S., *Social Psychology of the Work Organisation,* Tavistock Publications, London, 1966.

Taylor, B., 'Strategies for Planning', *Long Range Planning,* August 1975.

Thompson, E. J., 'Population Projections for Metropolitan Areas', *Greater London Intelligence Quarterly,* No. 28, September 1974.

Tibbitt, J. E., *The Social Work/Medicine Interface: A Review of Research,* Social Work Services Group, Scottish Education Department, 1975.

Towell, D., and Dartington, T., 'Encouraging innovations in hospital care', *Journal of Advance Nursing I,* 1976.

Townsend, P., 'Inequality and the Health Service', *The Lancet,* 15 June 1974.

Townsend, P., 'Area Deprivation Policies', *New Statesman,* 6 August 1976.

Trades Union Congress, *Industrial Democracy: Interim Report,* TUC, London, 1973.

Tudor Hart, J., 'The Inverse Care Law', *The Lancet,* 27 February 1971.

Vaizey, J. (ed.), *Whatever happened to equality?,* BBC, 1975.

Wadsworth, M. E. J., Butterfield, W. J. H., and Blaney, R., *Health and Sickness: The Choice of Treatment,* Tavistock, London, 1971.

Walker, K. F., 'Workers Participation in Management: Concepts and Reality' in B. Barrett, E. Rhodes and J. Beishon (eds.), *Industrial Relations and the Wider Society,* Collier-Macmillan, London, 1975.

Wilkes, E., 'Unlimited Demand—limited resources', *The Hospital and Health Services Review,* August 1976.

Wilson, M., *Health is for People,* Darton, Longman and Todd, London, 1975.

Woolf, M., *Family Intentions,* HMSO, 1972.

Wolman, D. M., 'Quality Control and the Community Physician in England: An American Perspective', *International Journal of Health Services,* 6(1), 1976.

Woolf, M., and Pegden, S., *Families Five Years On,* HMSO, 1976.

Zborowski, M., 'Cultural Components in Response to Pain', *Journal of*

Social Issues, 8, 16, 1952.

Zola, I. K., 'Culture and Symptoms: An Analysis of Patients Presenting Complaints', *American Sociological Review,* 31, 5, 1960.

Zola, I. K., 'Illness Behaviour of the Working Class' in A. Shostak and W. Gomberg (eds.), *Blue Collar World: Studies of the American Worker,* Prentice-Hall, Englewood Cliffs, New Jersey, 1964.

Zola, I. K., 'Medicine as an Institution of Social Control', *Sociological Review,* 20, 3, November 1972.

Official Documents and Reports

Internal Administration of Hospitals, Central Health Services Council (Bradbeer Report), 1954.

Report on the Grading Structure of Administrative and Clerical Staff in the Hospital Service (Hall Report), 1957.

Report of Joint Working Party on the Medical Staffing Structure in the Hospital Service (Platt Report), Ministry of Health, 1961.

Accident and Emergency Services (Platt Report), Central Health Services Council, 1962.

The Field of Work of the Family Doctor (Gillie Report), Ministry of Health, 1963.

Report of the Committee on Senior Nursing Staff Structure (Salmon Report), 1966.

Report of the Committee on Hospital Supplies Organisation (Hunt Report), 1966.

Administrative Practice of Hospital Boards in Scotland (Farquharson-Lang Report), Scottish Health Services Council, 1966.

First Report of the Joint Working Party on the Organisation of Medical Work in Hospitals (Godber Report), Ministry of Health, 1967.

The Pay and Conditions of Manual Workers in Local Authorities, the National Health Service, Gas and Water Supply, National Board for Prices and Incomes Report No. 29, 1967.

Report of the Committee on Hospital, Scientific and Technical Services (Zuckerman Report), 1968

Payment by Results System, National Board for Prices and Incomes Report No. 65, 1968.

Green Paper on the Administrative Structure of the Medical and Related Services in England and Wales, Ministry of Health, 1968.

The Royal Commission on Medical Education, 1965-1968 (Todd Report), 1968.

The Royal Commission on Trade Unions and Employers' Associations,

1965-1968 (Donovan Report), Cmnd. 3623, 1968.

Consumer Consultative Machinery in the Nationalised Industries, Report by the Consumer Council, 1968.

Report of the Committee of Inquiry into Allegations of Ill-Treatment of Patients and Other Irregularities at the Ely Hospital, Cardiff, Cmnd. 3975, 1969.

Report of the Working Party on the Responsibilities of the Consultant Grade (Godber Report), 1969.

Report of the Working Party on the Hospital Pharmaceutical Services (Noel Hall Report), 1970.

Report of the Farleigh Hospital Committee of Inquiry, Cmnd. 4557, 1971.

Relations with the Public: Second Report from the Select Committee on Nationalised Industries, 1971.

National Health Service Reorganisation: Consultative Document, DHSS, 1971.

National Health Service Reorganisation: England, Cmnd. 5055, DHSS, 1972.

Management Arrangements for the Reorganised National Health Service, (Grey Book), DHSS, 1972.

Report of the Working Party on Medical Administrators (Hunter Report), DHSS, 1972.

Population Projections 1973-2003, OPCS, 1972.

Report of the Committee of Inquiry into Whittingham Hospital, Cmnd. 4861, 1972.

Second Report of Joint Working Party on the Organisation of Medical Work in Hospitals (Godber Report), DHSS, 1972.

Report of the Committee on Hospital Complaints Procedure (Davies Report), 1973.

Accident and Emergency Services, Vols. I and II, Fourth Report of the Expenditure Committee of the House of Commons, 1974.

Report of the Committee of Inquiry into South Ockendon Hospital, HC24, 1974.

Democracy in the National Health Service, DHSS, 1974.

Third Report of the Joint Working Party on the Organisation of Medical Work in Hospitals (Godber Report), DHSS, 1974.

Population Projections 1973-2003, OPCS, 1974.

A Joint Framework for Social Policy, Central Policy Review Staff, June 1975.

Report of the Committee of Inquiry into the Regulations of the Medical Profession (Merrison Report), 1975.

Accident and Emergency Services, Government Observations on the Fourth Report of the Employment and Social Services Sub-Committee of the Expenditure Committee, Cmnd. 5886, DHSS, 1975.

Better Services for the Mentally Ill, Cmnd. 6233, 1975.

Allocations to Regions in 1976/77, The First Interim Report of the Resource Allocation Working Party, DHSS, August 1975.

Variant Population Projections, OPCS, 1975.

Public Expenditure to 1979-80, Cmnd. 6393, February 1976.

Priorities for Health and Personal Social Services in England: A Consultative Document, DHSS, April 1976.

Cash Limits on Public Expenditure, Cmnd. 6440, April 1976.

Local Government Finance: Report by the Committee of Inquiry (Layfield Committee), Cmnd. 6453, May 1976.

Consumers and the Nationalised Industries: Report of the National Consumer Council, 1976.

Sharing Resources for Health in England, Report of the Resource Allocation Working Party, DHSS, September 1976.

INDEX